HANDREADING

Founded by C. K. Ogden

The International Library of Psychology

INDIVIDUAL DIFFERENCES
In 21 Volumes

I	The Practice and Theory of Individual Psychology	*Adler*
II	The Neurotic Constitution	*Adler*
III	Duality	*Bradley*
IV	Problems of Personality	*Campbell et al*
V	An Introduction to Individual Psychology	*Dreikurs*
VI	The Psychology of Alfred Adler and the Development of the Child	*Ganz*
VII	Personality	*Gordon*
VIII	The Art of Interrogation	*Hamilton*
IX	Appraising Personality	*Harrower*
X	Physique and Character	*Kretschmer*
XI	The Psychology of Men of Genius	*Kretschmer*
XII	Handreading	*Laffan*
XIII	On Shame and the Search for Identity	*Lynd*
XIV	A B C of Adler's Psychology	*Mairet*
XV	Alfred Adler: Problems of Neurosis	*Mairet*
XVI	Principles of Experimental Psychology	*Piéron*
XVII	The Psychology of Character	*Roback*
XVIII	The Hands of Children	*Spier*
XIX	The Nature of Intelligence	*Thurstone*
XX	Alfred Adler: The Pattern of Life	*Wolfe*
XXI	The Psychology of Intelligence and Will	*Wyatt*

HANDREADING

A Study of Character and Personality

M N LAFFAN

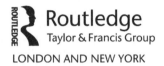

Routledge
Taylor & Francis Group

LONDON AND NEW YORK

First published in 1932 by
Kegan Paul, Trench, Trubner & Co., Ltd.
2 Park Square, Milton Park, Abingdon, Oxfordshire OX14 4RN
711 Third Avenue, New York, NY 10017

First issued in paperback 2014

Routledge is an imprint of the Taylor and Francis Group, an informa business

British Library Cataloguing in Publication Data
A CIP catalogue record for this book
is available from the British Library

Handreading
ISBN 978-0415-21062-1
Individual Differences: 21 Volumes
ISBN 0415-21130-1
The International Library of Psychology: 204 Volumes
ISBN 0415-19132-7

ISBN 13: 978-1-138-87541-8 (pbk)
ISBN 13: 978-0-415-21062-1 (hbk)

CONTENTS

CHAPTER   PAGE

I.   THEORIES - - - - - - 1

II.   METHOD - - - - - - 19

III.   THE LINE OF INSTINCT OR "LIFE LINE" - - - - - - 33

IV.   THE LINE OF REASON OR "HEAD LINE" - - - - - - 42

V.   THE LINE OF INTUITION OR "HEART LINE" - - - - - - 53

VI.   THE THUMB - - - - - 58

VII.   THE INDEX FINGER - - - - 66

VIII.   THE OTHER FINGERS - - - 72

IX.   IMAGINATION - - - - - 76

X.   THE SHAPE OF THE HAND - - 80

XI.   THE LINE OF FATE - - - - 88

XII.   THE LINE OF PERSONALITY - - 97

XIII.   HEALTH AND OTHER LINES - - 104

XIV.   SQUARES, STARS AND CROSSES - 110

XV.   CONCLUSION - - - - - 118

LIST OF ILLUSTRATIONS

Plate   *Facing page*

I. HAND OF A GIRL TWELVE YEARS OLD - 14

II. THE SAME HAND FOURTEEN YEARS LATER, SHOWING CHANGED POSITION OF REASON LINE AND IMPROVED INSTINCT - - - 14

III. DIAGRAM SHOWING PARTS OF THE PALM WHICH REPRESENT INSTINCT AND IMAGINATION: ALSO THE POSITION OF THE LINE OF CLAIRVOYANCE AND THE LINES OF INFLUENCE AND THE PHALANGES OF THE THUMB - - - 22

IV. HAND OF ACTIVE TYPE WITH STRONG INSTINCT LINE AND A LINE OF INITIATIVE - - 34

V. HAND OF ELEMENTARY TYPE - - - 44

VI. HAND OF IDEALISTIC TYPE WITH STRONG LINE OF REASON - - - - - - 44

VII. HAND WITH GOOD INTUITION LINE FOR BUSINESS AFFAIRS: ALSO POLITICAL ABILITY - - 54

VIII. HAND OF ARTIST WITH CREATIVE INTUITION - 54

IX. HAND OF PAINTER WITH STRONG IMAGINATION AND ARTISTIC TALENT - - - - 74

X. THE SAME HAND A YEAR LATER SHOWING IMPROVED PERSONALITY LINE AND CREATIVE POWER - - - - - - - 74

XI. HAND WITH CLEAR LINES OF FATE AND PERSONALITY. DATES ARE INDICATED BY POINTS 88

XII. HAND SHOWING THE LINES OF HEALTH, OF MARRIAGE, OF SENSITIVENESS, AND THE MYSTIC CROSS - - - - - 106

vii

LIST OF ILLUSTRATIONS

Plate   Facing Page

CHAPTER I

THE study of Personality throws a wide net over many subjects, and to-day the markings of the human hand are engaging the interest of practical minds. For many years I have been observing handmarkings as an index to character and personality, and I am convinced that if the study of the hand were developed in a scientific way it would prove a valuable aid to the understanding of " the capacities, dispositions and tendencies that make up the whole mind."[1] Moreover, through handreading the individual may be helped to a clearer knowledge of his powers and limitations than would otherwise be possible.

The study of the shape and lines of the hand has not yet received scientific treatment, partly because of the difficulty of extricating the empirical evidence from the confused systems of palmistry, and its association with fortune telling or divination. But some empirical

[1] McDougall, *The Group Mind.*

evidence of the correlation of handmarkings with mental characteristics, though it is admittedly extremely meagre, hypothetical, fragmentary, and difficult of access, does exist.

I have had the opportunity of observing the hands of many interesting individuals, some of them from time to time during a course of years. This enabled me to watch the changes in the lines, and their relation to the development of the mind. I do not however claim to have evolved a proper system, or to have ascertained the exact truth regarding handmarkings ; but merely to have accumulated, from my observation of hands and the study of books on palmistry and modern psychology, sufficient data to form a basis for the collection of new evidence of the correlation of handmarkings and mental characteristics. If I appear over-dogmatic in my statements in this book, it is merely for the purpose of a clear exposition.

In ancient times, handreading was honoured and practised by the great races of ´mankind. Chaldeans, Indians, Egyptians, Hebrews, Arabs, and notably the Greeks and Romans, esteemed the study of the hand a definite science ; Aristotle wrote a great deal concerning it in his *History of Animals,* and the historian Josephus is said to describe Cæsar as such an expert hand-reader that having once seen a man's hands he could not be deceived as to his pretensions.

Though generally attributed to the Hindus, the exact origin of palmistry is uncertain. In *La Psychologie de la Main* (a modern book described in the preface by Professor Charles Richet[1] as " une œuvre faite d'originalité et de l'érudition ") the late Dr. Vaschide[2] discusses the possibility of handreading having developed apart from astrology. He considers that this is unlikely, but says that in the opinion of some writers, and particularly of Alfred Lehmann,[3] the Danish psychologist, palmistry originated as an independent study among the Bohemians and Tartars. Dr. Vaschide adds that this view is tenable " especially as the history of chiromancy has not yet been written."

The origin of Palmistry among nomadic tribes may easily be imagined. Seated round their camp fires, holding up their hands to the blaze, they would have noticed the lines across their

[1] Professeur à la Faculté de Médecine de Paris, membre de l'Académie des Sciences et de l'Académie de Médecine, professeur de physiologie, 1887.

[2] Directeur-adjoint du Laboratoire de Psychologie Pathologique de l'Ecole des Hautes-Etudes, Paris, 1874-1907.

[3] Professor of the University of Copenhagen, 1895-1903, author of several books on philosophy and psychology.

companions' palms. Their curiosity would have been aroused by the likeness and unlikeness of the hands themselves, and the lines across them. They would have seen that their men of action mostly had square hands and strong lines round the thumb (which we call now the line of Instinct); that their wise men, whose counsel was valued, all had long hands and a strong middle line across the palm (the line of Reason). Poets, who sang to them of love and adventure, and their most magnetic women, had hands of a different type; fine, sensitive hands, the salient characteristic being the high line across the palm, which we call the line of Intuition. Maybe, too, they saw that those of their friends who had weak or broken lines often had accidents, sometimes even a violent death. It is easy to imagine how they looked at hands, and talked of the meanings of lines and marks, and so arrived at a generalized idea of the association of a certain sort of character with a particular shape of hand and position of the lines. They were, of course, prone to make signs and omens out of other and simpler associations, but with far less opportunity of checking the truth of the relationship, which they were apt to take for granted after one coincidence only, especially if it happened to suit their mood and purpose to do so. The meaning of handmarkings, however, would be compared and checked by communal discussion and observation, and the truth sifted from error more easily than it could be in the case of omens read in the flights of birds, the shape of the clouds, and other nature phenomena.

To gypsies and other nomads, the characters and emotions of individuals are the very stuff of life's interest and enjoyment, so that the hand-markings and their meanings would be of supreme value; and a competent handreader might acquire honour and fame. Knowledge of interpretations that they found were reliable would be a treasured possession, and carefully handed on to their descendants. But always there would be fresh empirical observation of hands and the meaning attached to the shape and lines, so that in time their significance would become an established tradition; and this would form a basis for the instinctive perceptions of their free uncultured minds.

About a hundred years ago, observation of hands took place in very different circumstances. A smart young French officer, proud of his shapely hands, noticed that at the receptions at a neighbouring château the particular friends of the hostess all had hands somewhat alike, and very different from those of her husband's friends. Madame loved art and poetry, Monsieur cared only for engineering affairs. From these observations, Monsieur le Capitaine d'Arpentigny[1] was impelled to investigate the meaning of the different shapes of the human hand, and he wrote a book which has been looked on as a classic by later writers.

Desbarolles,[2] the author of *Les Mystères de la Main*, who was a contemporary, quotes largely from d'Arpentigny's book, and Desbarolles may be called the " Father of Modern Palmistry." He did for the lines and marks what d'Arpentigny had done for the shape of the hand. He seems to have relied on the system expounded in the Kabala ; but he had an opportunity, during a long life, of studying the hands of the eminent men and women of France, and was alert to gather confirmation of his interpretation of the meaning of lines and marks.

In my own case, interest in handmarkings was aroused by the exact fulfilment of a palmist's prophecy to a friend that he would shortly have

[1] Stanislas d'Arpentigny, author of *Chirognomonie ou la Science de la Main*, Paris, 1856.
[2] Adrien Desbarolles, a famous French palmist, author of *Les Mystères de la Main*, Paris, 1859.

a very bad accident. Of course this might have been merely a coincidence, but his hand showed a curious formation ; for the primary lines were all three joined together, and in palmistry books this is said to be " a presage of misfortune." I could not find any other hands with this peculiar arrangement of the lines ; but I did find that any unusual shape or marking was significant of the character and mentality of the individuals in whose hands I found it. Moreover, my " readings " were often a very great help and enlightenment to people, both as to the nature of their minds and also how to deal with the problems of their lives. In the case of difficult children the help given was often of very great importance. Therefore I continued to study hands with the aid of Desbarolles' *Mystères de la Main* and " Cheiro's "[1] *Language of the Hand,* though I could not believe in their theories as to the cause of the lines, and in many respects found their methods inadequate and confused.

Most palmists attribute handmarkings to the influence of the stars, and the theory of some writers on Handreading is that " the astral fluid

---

[1] A famous palmist and seer. In 1900 celebrities of world renown were among " Cheiro's " clientèle. His books on Palmistry are in demand to-day.

7

flows in through the finger tips and causes the lines in the palm." Since astrology and palmistry were associated, astrological names were considered natural for parts of the hand and for the lines. It is however more practical and more scientific to think of the hand simply as an instrument of the mind, and of the marks and lines as a record of mental characteristics. Psychological science presents suitable names which we may borrow to assist in the understanding of the significance of the unusual formations which are frequently encountered. Moreover, it is an advantage that in discarding the names of ancient deities for parts of the hand, and substituting the name of the member itself or its significance only, the study is greatly simplified.

In the present state of our knowledge it is difficult to believe that the stars are intimately concerned with the chances and changes of our individual lives, so that if after numerous observations of hands we are convinced that there is a substratum of truth in the old systems of Palmistry, a new theory to account for the markings of the human hand is important and even necessary.

Unlike Astrology, Handreading is not dependent on occult knowledge or influence. Interpretation of the meaning of the shape and the lines of the hand is based on observations that can be compared and have to a certain extent been verified. The work of the old writers provides a useful guide for its reconstruction as a modern study ; but a revision of method and nomenclature is necessary as well as observation and the careful tabulation of results.

So far as I know, however, nothing of the sort has yet been attempted. Authors of books on the subject have been content to rely almost entirely on the old systems ; and, though they add remarks on their own experience and the truth of their predictions, these are not in the nature of evidence for the truth of Handreading.

Psycho-analysts discovered that the ancient practice of interpretation of dreams had a valuable substratum of truth, and in the light of modern knowledge they have constructed a system by which they make use of dreams for their study of the human mind, more especially the unconscious urges and motives. The work of distinguished psycho-analysts has proved of great value both for the treatment of mental disease and also for knowledge of the nature and powers of the mind. Indeed, on the basis of an immense amount of observation, particularly of pathological cases, they have been able to construct an entire systematic psychology.

Handreading also badly needs scientific investigation and reconstruction. Though indirect, it is a much simpler study of the mind than psycho-analysis, since it deals with the objective indications which the lines of the hand give of the mental organisation as the basis of character and conduct. This, of course, is a postulate at present. It is also concerned more with the conscious development of the mind than with the discovery of the unconscious desires and hidden motives. Hence it is probably more useful for normal people as a guide to wise self-discipline and the understanding and education of their children.

It is obvious that every individual starts life with capacities and potentialities that differ, sometimes in kind and sometimes in degree, from those of every other individual. Can these capacities and potentialities be accurately deciphered from the shape and lines of the hand? Though this can only be fully proved by strict investigation, my own experience convinces me that they can—in other words the lines in the palm of the hand show the mental make-up and organisation or "life plan" of the individual.

Can a forecast of future events and changes of life be made from the lines in the palm ? So far as they depend on one's mental characteristics, I have had strong evidence that in a general degree they can ; but there is also evidence that conscious effort has some control over the lines themselves. I have often seen the lines in hands change—either develop or fade—as directed by the wishes and efforts of their owners. This possible growth of new or improving lines could soon be demonstrated in experimental work. Plates IX and X show the development of the line of Personality that took place within a year in the hand of an artist. Unusual success was achieved during this period and the age is approximately given by the line.

It is difficult to believe that the future can be confidently predicted ; for it seems impossible that the chances of life which come from outside influences can be foreseen, except perhaps in those rare cases where the mind has an unconscious foreknowledge of the future. Where this exists it may possibly be apprehended by a Handreader (or seer of any sort) who has a gift of clairvoyance or telepathy[1] ; and this I think might account for many of the successful prophecies of future events that are quoted by clairvoyants of all kinds. But the successful prophecies are in reality exceedingly rare compared with the mass of unsuccessful and unrecorded ones. Owing to this uncertainty, described by Hegel as " the dim and turbid vision of clairvoyance," its practical utility is more than doubtful, though its fascination is very great.

The ancient Seers or " Occult Masters " were mostly wise men of great experience, the philosophers and psychologists of their time. Nowadays practical training and intellectual development may subordinate the telepathic or clairvoyant powers ; and the people who possess and use them are generally speaking not trained in scientific subjects or medical knowledge.

The prophetic power of the mind is mysterious and difficult to examine. There seem to be two distinct methods of gaining knowledge that are beyond our conscious grasp ; one an instinctive

[1] McDougall, in *An Outline of Abnormal Psychology* (page 517), defines telepathy as " the direct communication of mind with mind without the use of sense perception." In *Body and Mind* (page 349) he writes : " I cannot attempt to present here the evidence for the reality of telepathy. It must suffice to say that it is of such a nature as to compel the assent of any competent person who studies it impartially."

apprehension of conditions and thoughts, in the nature of telepathy, which animals apparently share in some degree; the other intuitive and visionary, best obtained by minds developed through spiritual or mental effort.

It is important to discriminate between knowledge that can be gained by a wise synthesis of the indications of the mental life given by the shape and lines of the hand, and knowledge of the personality, its conditions and problems, that the Handreader may be able to reach by clairvoyance or by telepathy. Though often of greater interest, and possibly even greater value for the individual, knowledge so gained is not so reliable as the interpretation of handmarkings. So many factors are involved that cannot be controlled, and the results cannot be analysed or tabulated. Accordingly, though these gifts may have their place and value, they are of no assistance in a scientific examination of Handreading.

When I first studied hands I found that ideas and impressions frequently drifted into my mind for which I could find no justification in the handmarkings; but they were generally true, more personal, and more exciting than conclusions based on the markings of the hand. By ignoring these impressions my " readings " were rendered somewhat dull compared to those of professional palmists ; but I firmly repressed all unconsciously formed opinions, as they gave me no evidence of the real meaning of the hand-markings which I was bent on discovering. There seems no reason, however, why the clairvoyant perceptions of the Handreader should not be taken into account, once the study of the hand has been established on a rational basis.

The reputation of a doctor depends not only on his medical knowledge and skill, but also on his powers of sympathy and insight, which give him a more complete and intimate knowledge of his patients than could be acquired by consideration of their symptoms alone. Therefore it would be unreasonable to deny the value of such powers of insight in connection with the work of Handreading. But in the first place the knowledge of the meaning to be attached to the lines and shape of the hand, and the ability to weigh the value of the contrasting mental qualities which are indicated should be considered of fundamental importance. For the practice of Handreading we assume that there is a correlation between mental characters and parts of the hand—which is the instrument of the brain—and that the pre-natal growth of the members and lines of the hand

PLATE 1

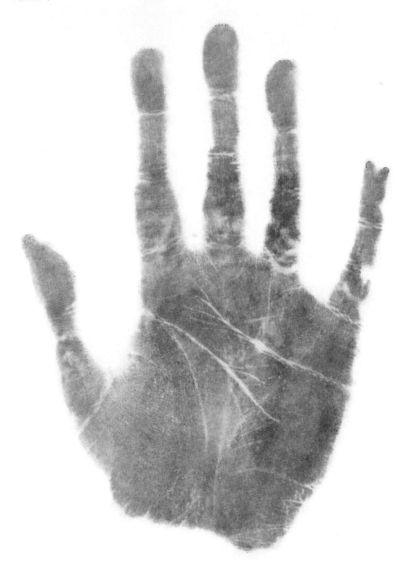

The hand of a girl twelve years old, showing the Reason line joined to the Instinct line. The latter is somewhat short

[face Plate II, after p. 14

PLATE II

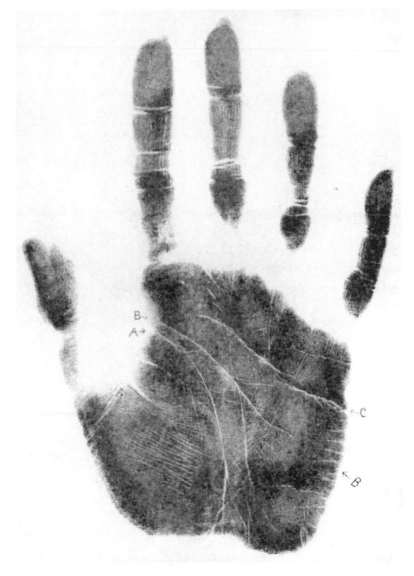

A. The Instinct line
B. The Reason line
C. The Intuition line

The same hand as Plate 1, but fourteen years later. The lines of Instinct and of Reason, which were joined together at twelve years old, are now separated. The mind has gained independence and intellectual power. The Instinct line has grown longer, showing an improved constitution

[face Plate I

took place in close correspondence with the formation of the brain, its powers and potentialities, and can be taken as in some degree representing the nature of the mind. Only careful and accurate observation can affirm or disprove that this correspondence exists and continues in the life of the individual.

I am told that hands are marked, and also move, before birth. Certainly when babies are born their hands are often heavily lined or creased. I have noticed that as time goes on and the little hands are less often closely folded, some of the lines disappear, and all become less deeply marked. The primary lines change much less than the secondary ones. Very rarely is there such an alteration in position of a primary line as is shown in Plates I and II. Plate I is the handprint of a girl of twelve, showing the Reason line joined to the Instinct line. Plate II shows that at twenty-five years of age the two lines have become separated. The Reason line has moved to a position higher in the hand, indicating more independence of the intellectual capacity. This development coincided with the necessity of controlling a large country house owing to the untimely death of the young girl's mother.

The lines of the hands seem to be partly caused

by the contraction of muscles, which make folds or patterns in the skin. I understand that these muscles are innervated by efferent neurones having their origin in the brain; and I am told that when, through some accident or disease, cortical control is interfered with, violent movements of the limbs and undisciplined emotions result. But the actual physiological explanation of the primary lines or folds across the palm is a matter for scientific investigation. The only scientific book I have come across that gives more than a cursory glance at the ancient study of Palmistry is *La Psychologie de la Main* by Dr. Vaschide; in which he says " Il est remarquable que ces grandes plis, considérés comme les plus importants par les chiromanciennes, aient des rapports intimes avec des salies musculaires, avec des articulations métacarpiennes, avec des insertions musculaires, aponévrotiques ou tendineuses " (page 476). If satisfactory evidence could be collected that the three folds across the palm are definitely correlated with the faculties of Instinct, Reason, and Intuition, physiologists and psychologists might be encouraged to further research.

The collection of evidence for the correlation of the shape and lines of the hand with certain mental characteristics is the first necessary step towards a definite science of Handreading. If the study can be established on a satisfactory basis it promises to be valuable in many directions, more especially to those individuals who wish to understand, and develop to the highest possible point, the capacities of their minds.

The mystery that fascinated human minds in the past is still with us in another form. We no longer think that in the will of the Gods, or influences of the stars, lies the origin of our fate. But within the mind there are depths as mysterious and unfathomable, desires and urges as imperious, as the will of the Gods that men imagined to be the masters of their destiny ; and they seem as uncontrollable. The change is one of location only. Not above and beyond, but within, lies the mysterious world of destiny. It is not easy to examine this world of the innermost self, indeed it seems as far removed as the occult powers from the experience of everyday life.

It is, of course, possible that the earlier faith is nearer the truth, that our minds are but the instruments of higher beings or cosmic forces driving us to express ourselves according to their will, and that the depth of our being does not originate the urges and desires that drive us.

C

Intellect and will are, however, improving as instruments for dealing with these promptings, whatever their origin may be ; and in the development of our conscious knowledge and power lies the greatest promise both for the happiness of the individual and also for the fulfilment of the dream of human progress.

CHAPTER II

METHOD

THE study of the hand is composed of two parts—the study of the lines and the study of the shape; for Handreading a knowledge of both is necessary.

Dr. Vaschide says, " According to the harmony that exists between the palm and the fingers one may presume the mental and physical equilibrium of the individual. The palm represents the personal faculties, the subjective elements of the brain, the individual elements characteristic of the mentality and of the greater or less resistance of the physical and moral health. The fingers indicate the expression, the form which is given to the thought, and from the physical point of view what is called in the usual language of palmists the atavistic laws of the temperament. They personify, in other words, the elegance, the artistic sense, etc. . . . the different forms of the psycho-physical temperament, act, or agitation, the act of prehension, of contact."[1]

[1] *La Psychologie de la Main*, page 63.

If this be so, a quick glance both at the shape and the lines of each hand is advisable in order to form a rough estimate of the quality of the mind as a whole before studying the significance of each part separately.

Handreaders are generally advised to consider first the shape or the type of hand. I think, however, that the primary lines which show the intellectual capacities are of first importance. These capacities may be counteracted to some extent by abnormal weakness of disposition, but they are the ruling factors in the development of the mind.

Students are apt to find books on Handreading very confusing, owing to so many different meanings being more or less arbitrarily attributed to one part or line of the hand ; even Desbarolles and " Cheiro " err in this respect. For instance, the thumb is said by its three divisions to indicate not only the will, the judgment, and the love disposition of the individual, but also various other qualities and tastes. A strong thumb might be likely to " go with " these other qualities ; but their possession should be learnt from the parts or the lines of the hand which specially signify them. Assuming positive correlation, each line, or part, should be given its own special meaning only.

METHOD

The order of notation I advise is :

1st.   The three Primary Lines.
      Instinct, Reason, Intuition (or Life, Head, Heart of the old systems).

2nd. The Thumb.
      The three divisions representing the power of the Will, of Judgment, and of Love.

3rd.   The Index Finger and Base.
      Power or lack of Ambition, Leadership, Creativeness.

4th.   The Other Fingers and Bases.
      Dispositions and Tastes.

5th.   Base of hand, the Hypothenar Eminence.
      Power of Imagination.

6th.   Shape of the Hand.
      Tendencies and Temperament.

7th.   Secondary or Upright Lines.
      The clash between the Personality and the Environment.

8th.   Other Lines.
      Health, Marriage, etc.

9th.   Squares, Crosses, and Stars.
      Special activities and possible events.

Unusual or abnormal features will be quickly noted in the preliminary survey of the hand as a whole ; and it is very important to bear in mind

PLATE III

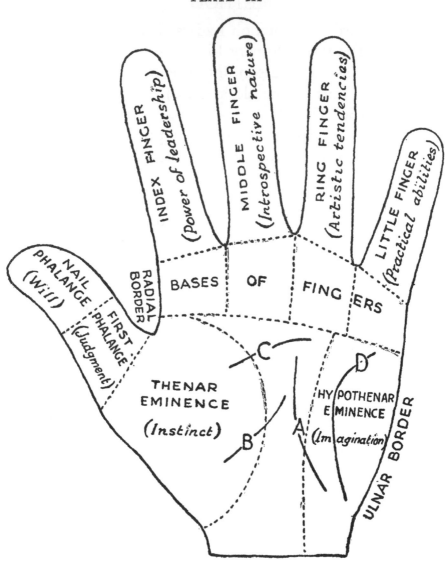

DIAGRAM SHOWING THE PARTS OF THE PALM WHICH REPRESENT THE INSTINCTS AND THE IMAGINATION, ALSO THE POSITION OF THE LINE OF CLAIRVOYANCE AND THE LINES OF INFLUENCE, AND THE PHALANGES OF THE THUMB.

A—Line of Happy Influence.   C—Line of Adverse Influence.
B—Line of Sex Influence.   D—Line of Clairvoyance.

the significance of any strong or unusual marking thus noted during the subsequent more detailed examination of each member and line of the hand —more especially of those that are most detrimental to the use and development of capacities strongly indicated.

To learn how one indication qualifies another should be one of the first tasks of the student. One is apt to overestimate capacities without realising a weakness that counteracts them.

A weak thumb closely set to the hand would discount the intellectual capacities, the tastes, the aptitudes, elsewhere shown, except those that are unusually good and strongly marked.

Badly shaped or crooked fingers, or the abnormal length of any one in particular, represent outstanding dispositions of the nature that may dominate the mind instead of serving it.

A flabby hand shows want of physical energy. Mental interest might counteract this ; and by a study of the lines the Handreader could suggest the best way to arouse mental activity and the subject most suitable for study, in which success might be achieved.

A thin hard hand represents a restless mind and would make the development of intellectual and artistic tastes difficult, but would not retard a practical or adventurous nature (shown by a strong line of Instinct).

A hand criss-crossed with many little lines—sometimes described as " a barbed wire entanglement " —indicates a mind distracted by thoughts and feelings, or a kind of nervous instability. This is especially the case when most of the lines come from the ball of the thumb and cross over the line of instinct into the middle of the palm. This indicates that all the little instinctive desires and urges, instead of being subordinated to higher activities, invade, and to some degree interfere with, the functioning of the intellectual faculties. With strength of will (shown by a moderately good thumb) these instinctive impulses might be controlled by concentrating on the special abilities of the mind which the Handreader may be able to point out. The condition might however be due to illness, and only temporary ; in such a case advice as to how best to improve the physical health by appropriate diet or mental occupation may be useful.

Hands that are exactly or very nearly alike indicate that the mind is a very stable and balanced one ; and, unless the stimulus of outside influences is strong, it is unlikely to develop in any particular direction. Any one outstanding capacity however would gain in significance by being observed in both hands.

Very flexible hands show an impressionable nature to which concentration or sustained purpose are difficult, owing to the ready response the mind makes to any and every distraction or demand for attention or sympathy. An exaggerated flexibility must be regarded as a qualification of the intellectual capacities and tastes.

When the primary lines are deep and strong but look like ruts rather than lines (Plate V), as is often the case in elementary or working-class hands, I think it indicates that the capacities of the mind are undeveloped or in abeyance. I was much puzzled at first by finding such good primary lines in the hands of monkeys and also of people whose intellects were not developed; but the condition best described as " empty " explains this. The lines are there in anticipation of function; and the thumbs are usually weak with this condition.

Hands that have no secondary or upright lines are difficult to read because they show a nature that lacks a definite plan, or pattern, which may be deciphered; but I do not think there is any evidence that the lack of lines forebodes an early death, as some writers claim; for I have seen the secondary lines develop in hands that at one time had none. But a plan, even though an unconscious one, would no doubt strengthen the hold on life of an individual who without a definite purpose might more easily succumb to an illness or disaster. Careful examination will generally disclose some small beginnings or incipient lines of personal development ; and I feel quite sure, from my own experience, that to direct the attention of the subject to these lines and their meanings is of very great importance. It helps the personality to develop, to recognise—as people generally do when the meaning of the line is pointed out—that they have some special gift or capacity that only requires effort to become established as a source of pleasure and profit. On the other hand, some fault or indulgence that is blocking the right development may be made perceptible. It is curious how ignorant individuals often are of the possibilities of their own minds.

The shape of the hand qualifies the lines. For instance, a very good line of reason would have a different significance in an elementary hand from that of a similar line in a philosophic type of hand.

There is a curious line sometimes termed the Mongol line, sometimes the Murderer's line. I think its significance depends almost entirely on the shape and other features of the hand. It is, roughly speaking, a line that combines the two primary lines of Reason and Intuition in one. In a hand showing a bad disposition (crooked fingers, etc.) this might indicate a mind prone to violent temper or brutal acts.

In a fine, well-shaped hand the line would indicate unusual strength of intellect. To call such an individual a murderer would be absurd. Ruthless he might be, but only when a situation demanded strong action.

Then there is the problem of the meaning of the difference between the two hands to be considered. " The left is the hand you are born with, the right is the hand you make," is the explanation given by all books on Palmistry. This is not quite satisfactory. At birth there are differences between the shape and markings of the two hands, and often very great ones. Moreover, the markings of both hands change during life.

My own observation led me to the hypothesis that we might consider the differences in the shape and lines of the two hands as due to differences in the organisation of the two cerebral hemispheres ; just as we know right- or left-handedness is dependent on this. Thus the hand governed by the stronger or better organised hemisphere becomes " the master hand."

Left-handed people are those whose best organised hemisphere is the right one, the motor neurones of which govern the left side of the body. Being the stronger so far as the hand is concerned, it refuses to let the right hand govern, and itself becomes " the master." Then the conscious development is shown by the lines and markings in the left hand.

Careful examination of the hands of several left-handed people convinced me that the reason of their left-handedness was the mental superiority shown by the left hand ; for the lines indicating the intellectual capacities were in every case so much better and stronger than those in the right.

Consideration of slight differences in the case of right-handed people confirmed this hypothesis. Lines or marks in the left hand only showed underlying or semi-conscious powers—or tastes. Ambidexterity would be a good test, but I have not seen a case where it was complete. Persons who can use both hands almost equally well are rare, but in one or two cases I have seen, the markings, though not exactly alike in each hand, were of nearly equal value, which is unusual.

Ordinarily, the two hands do not differ very much. When there is a great difference there is a problem for the Handreader—and generally speaking for the person whose hands show such difference also—to work out. In two or three cases of very marked difference, amounting almost to a dual personality, the subject has agreed with this analysis. Though admittedly not sufficiently numerous to prove such a theory, I have never personally come across a case that did not support this hypothesis of the difference between the two hands.

I had an interesting experience of the difference between the two hands in the early days of my study, at a time when I still used the old formula " The left is the hand you are born with, the right is the hand you make." I was visiting the home of a very clever man whose hands I was most anxious to see. I had first of course to ask if I might read his wife's hands, though from her very direct and personal questions immediately we met as to my soul's salvation, I knew her to be suffering from religious mania. To my amazement her right hand had quite good normal lines ; it was the left hand that had the over-developed eminence of Imagination, the sloping line of Reason and stiff close-set thumb. These features being together with no sign of artistic tastes might well denote fanaticism.

I thought that Palmistry was very certainly wrong, but kept to its dogmas as I had determined I would always do, no matter what I thought. I told her that she had been born with an egotistical disposition and a morbid imagination, but that she had made herself a sensible and sympathetic woman. I emphasized and praised this development, though from what I knew of the lady it did not fit the facts. When I had finished the reading, her brother-in-law asked :

" What difference would it make if the person was left-handed ? "

" Oh, in that case, according to Palmistry, it would exactly reverse things ; the right hand would then represent what you were born, the left what you had made yourself," I replied. I noticed his amused expression as I answered his question. Then he said with slightly malicious emphasis :

" My sister-in-law *is* left-handed."

It was a difficult situation for me and I felt the tense silence of the other members of the party. But luckily the lady herself was very pleased with the reading and did not seem to realise all that this reversal meant.

Later on, when I had evolved my own interpretation of the difference between the two hands, I saw that this case supported my hypothesis.

The old formula would have implied that the lady had developed her abnormal dispositions herself, whereas I felt sure that such a great change could not have been brought about by conscious effort. The difference in the hands must have been there at birth. Using the left hand most would, I imagine, give greater power to the faculties represented by its abnormal formations. As the right hand was less used for conscious purposes, the better though weaker qualities it represented would belong only to the secondary self. A friend who knew her well confirmed this interpretation. The lady, she said, possessed two natures or personalities, one that of an intolerant bigot, the other a kind and sympathetic woman. Ordinarily, the narrow-minded self held sway, but in any great trouble or crisis the sympathetic woman emerged.

I have never seen any other person's hands differ so greatly as this lady's; but I have frequently come across cases in which the left hand pointed to some superior mental quality. The individual generally has a feeling of some latent power or knowledge he possesses but cannot reach. For this reason I think the left hand represents the less conscious or secondary self. It seems that in moments of great excitement or mental strain this underlying and elusive self is more available. The individual feels that he is obtaining the use of his latent power, even if its nature is not fully grasped. This is more especially the case if the emotional moment occurs after a period of solitude.

Several people with unusually different hands have told me that listening to good music gave them the feeling of being wholly, though somewhat dreamily, aware of a deeper self. This they feel as a definite enhancement of their personality which continues for some time and enables them to do more successful work.

The method and hypothesis I have tried to explain have proved satisfactory at least in my own experience, but this has naturally been limited ; and they need to be tested on a larger scale and by workers trained in scientific method. I make no claim that my work may be found more than merely suggestive. My hope is that it may provide a fresh starting point for a full investigation of the meaning of the shape and the markings of the hand.

CHAPTER III

THE lowest in the hand of the three primary lines skirts the ball of the thumb and so encloses the portion of the hand that seems to be correlated with the instinctive dispositions of the mind. To call this the Instinct line instead of the Life line—as it is named in the old systems—indicates what in my opinion is the particular capacity that it represents.

Roughly speaking, the impulses and actions that take place without our conscious efforts or direction may be termed instinctive, as well as the vital processes such as breathing, heart-beat, digestion, etc., which are necessary to life. And we shall find that when the line of Instinct is short, weakly marked, or broken, the vegetative and instinctive life is defective, injured or impoverished.

I am convinced that it is very false to predict and wrong to foretell early death because the line is short. It is wise to point out that there is probably some weakness of physical or instinctive force, and to advise that special care be taken in building up the constitution. No one can say that because the line is short now it will still be short in one year's time or longer.

I have personally not been able to observe such a growth of the line of Instinct ; but it is clearly shown in Plates I and II as having taken place, and I have seen equally great changes take place in other lines. Nor do I think it right to infer a long life because the line of Instinct is long and good. Danger to life may arise from other causes than the weakness of the nutritive and instinctive powers.

We now know enough of the potency of suggestion to realise the danger of putting an idea into the mind, more especially with the authoritative force of an accepted prediction given with all the prestige of a person in whom the subject has faith. But to say to the individual :— "You must build up your vitality to meet a possible weakness, or crisis at such an age" might be the means of saving his life. To be aware of the possibility of a future danger may be the means of averting it ; a little extra care for general health might improve the constitution,

PLATE IV

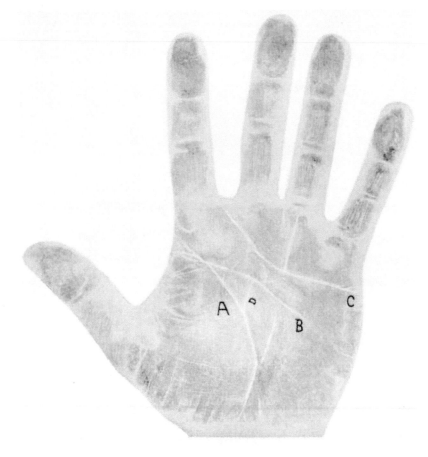

A. The Instinct line
B. The Reason line
C. The Intuition line
D. A line of Initiative

A man of action is shown by strong Instinct line. The greater width across the
base of the hand, denotes an enterprising nature

and the Instinct line grow stronger in consequence.

The line of Instinct commences on the border of the hand under the index finger. The best position is when it begins half way between the thumb and index finger, thus equally dividing the two parts which represent respectively intellectual pride and the combative instinct. The latter is indicated by what Palmists call the " Mount of Mars." This is the portion that is *inside* the Instinct line. The part *above* the line forms the base of the index finger and indicates, according to the lines and type of hand, either creative power, or pride, or ambition.

A strong clear line of Instinct sweeping well out into the hand indicates a man of action, Plate IV. This does not mean that the subject cannot be also a man of thought ; but if the line is stronger in every way than the other two primary lines, action—which demands a quick instinctive response to circumstances—would be the mode of expression best suited to the personality.

A line keeping close to the thumb would be a bad sign on an elementary hand, because the person showing this feature would need the stimulus of an emotional disposition. In a well-shaped, cultured hand in which the other lines are strongly marked, it would only indicate that the intellect had but little interference from instinctive impulses. Desbarolles is of the opinion that a line rising from high on the base of the index finger indicates an ambitious nature that nearly always succeeds in the " conquest of honours, ribbons and decorations, and high dignities." I have not come across such a line.

A double line, Desbarolles says, " is the luxury of existence." It seems to me likely to indicate a good constitution and unusual strength of the power of the vegetative and instinctive faculties, Plate VI. In the old terminology, the sister line is called the line of Mars, and is said in a woman's hand to signify success in love, and in a man's, success in warfare. I should call it the line of Vitality. I have seen it in the hands of successful actors and actresses, and frequently in the hands of those with a taste and desire for the stage ; but it seems likely to indicate the vitality and instinctive power which some possess of affecting other people ; a power necessary to support a dramatic career, rather than the career itself.

The line of Instinct joined to the two other primary lines is commonly said to be a " presage of misfortune." This will be dealt with later on.

From my experience I think it is undoubtedly true.

The line joined for some distance to the line we call that of Reason is said by Desbarolles to mean " timidity, excessive and insurmountable self-distrust " ; which, he adds, is a disease. As it is a very common formation, I have studied it a good deal and have come to the conclusion that the simple explanation is that the two lines being joined in an ordinary hand indicates that Reason is subordinated to Instinct ; the individual does not make efforts to reason things out logically, but acts almost entirely by instinct.

If this line is good, all is well. There does not seem much timidity in the actions or assertions of such people ; as a rule they are, so to speak, cocksure. It is only when the line of Instinct is weak that want of self-confidence appears ; and unless the intellectual lines of Reason and Intuition are good, this may lead to indecision and failure. It would seem that either Instinct or Reason must rule and direct thought and action if the individual is to achieve a strong personality.

The line when broken indicates some great change in life. If the new part of the line begins before the old leaves off, the change would be to better conditions. The break may be caused by illness or by some event such as travel, or a great shock. I have never seen such a break in a hand without finding it was true in the past that such a change had occurred at the time indicated; but I have never seen it as a future event.

A chained line indicates poor health either from organic disease or nervous debility.

Little lines leading down from this line show troubles or loss of strength. These I have seen in the " future " part of the line; and they have truly indicated a coming weakness, which eventually developed.

Little lines rising from the line indicate increasing health and well-being.

Islands in the line are signs of grave trouble caused sometimes by disgrace or a time of great strain; this I have always found accurate when interpreted to indicate a past event.

Small lines continually crossing the line from the base of the thumb, but not going far into the hand, indicate that desires, worries, or the tensions of life preoccupy the mind, and generally speaking cause unhappiness or a bad state of " nerves." Religious thought and practice can take the mind to higher levels, but where this is not congenial (this is sometimes only because it has not been tried), artistic, or scientific, or business interests may be cultivated and provide an antidote. Some sort of sublimation is necessary. Certainly the mind must be diverted from dwelling on instinctive conditions that cannot be controlled. A religious, moral, social, or intellectual interest is best, as it is of lasting value ; and most minds are capable of creating it in some form. If not, however, action or doing something definite is the only cure or alleviation.

When a strong line crosses the Instinct line and goes far into the palm and also crosses the secondary lines with a downward slope, it signifies a bad influence, generally of someone of the opposite sex, which affects the life adversely, Plate IIIc. If, however, the line rises and goes up the hand to the base of any of the fingers, the influence is likely to be helpful.

I have often seen these lines come and go in hands that I have been able to observe constantly, and they have always proved to be true indications. A warning of a growing influence might be useful ; but what Desbarolles calls " amours qui détruisent la destinée " are obsessions difficult to combat.

Little black spots on the line I have often seen as true indications of operations performed, or great nervous shocks experienced, in the past. I have never seen them in a position in which they might be taken to indicate future events.

Crosses on the line I have not seen. Desbarolles calls them a sign of mortal injury.

A line with a small cross on it is said by the same author to indicate a lawsuit. I have never however seen one.

Squares on or by the line I have very often observed, especially on the hands of soldiers. They are supposed to be signs of " preservation from danger." Where I have personally seen such squares this interpretation has been verified by the statements of the subject. When the square covers a thin or broken portion of the line, the " preservation " is from an illness.

When the line forks at the end, Desbarolles says it is a menace of weakness and loss of mental power in old age. " Cheiro," however, says it indicates a change to a new country from the one of birth. It might however be a new country of the mind. Thus a doctor or lawyer who took up agriculture as an offset to professional work might have the divided line, or a woman hitherto concerned chiefly with home life who took up philanthropic or political work. The forked line implies, I think, the expenditure of instinctive energy in two different directions.

The colour and width of the line give a good idea of the general health and strength. A pink, fairly broad line is the best. When red and deep it shows a brusque or turbulent nature ; when pale and thin a melancholy or weak one.

There are very important lines that rise from the line of Instinct itself ; they are said by all Palmists to signify " Increases won by personal merit," Plate IV. I have very often seen these lines truly indicating the time when the individual launched out " on his own," so to speak. It is an instinctive push of the whole nature towards its own ends ; and accordingly I prefer to call them lines of Initiative and not " a continuation of the Fate line " as they are generally termed. If seen rising from a " future " part of the line they would indicate the psychological moment for action ; and it might greatly help an individual to be aware of such a favourable sign.

CHAPTER IV

THE LINE OF REASON OR " HEAD LINE "

THE middle primary line is called by Palmists the line of " Head," but this is the name of a portion of the body and not of a function of the brain or of any mental character. Unless we recognise the precise capacity the line represents it is difficult to determine the meaning of the different positions in which it is constantly found in the palm. The power of Reason seems really to be what is meant by the word head, as when we speak of a man having " a good head on his shoulders " ; I found Reason as the significance of the line very satisfactory and was confirmed in the use of this term by reading that Sir Charles Sherrington in his presidential address to the British Association in 1922 described the mind of man as " actuated by instinct but instrumented with reason."

The lines of " Head " and " Heart " are both generally said to begin on or near the base of the index finger. But in that case one line would be beginning at its thinnest, the other at its thickest end. It would seem best to regard the Reason line, like the line of Intuition, as beginning at its thinnest end. I am here assuming a correlation between the imaginative power of the mind and the part of the hand called the hypothenar eminence; hence Reason would be said to begin in imagination. This agrees well enough with what we know of the faculty of Reason. First sensations and perceptions, next images, and then thoughts and ideas about them, which sometimes end in creative work, the power for which is shown by the base of the index finger to which the line of Reason tends.

A long, straight and clear line across the centre of the palm indicates a good logical reason, and, it is said, also a good memory.

A line beginning low on the palm and sloping up towards the base of the index finger indicates that the reasoning power is of an imaginative order; and if the ring finger, and especially its base, is well developed, this is likely to be used for expression in art; or, in a practical hand, for science, business, or other affairs of life. Where there are no special gifts for expression, such a line may indicate great independence of thought, tending to over self-confidence.

Ending on the very centre of the base of the index finger a strong line in a good hand indicates creativeness or an aptitude for making new forms, Plate VI. What these might be would depend on the nature of the mind as a whole. Individuals with fine intellects would create new ideas or forms of thought. A more practical mind would invent new machines. A woman with an elementary hand might be a good cook and would then invent new dishes. The creative line shows the capacity of the mind for forming new ideas or things ; the way in which this power will be used must be deciphered from other parts of the hand.

A good line that begins with a fork is said by " Cheiro " to promise literary talent. Desbarolles says it indicates deceit or " une manière de voir complètement fausse." It may, I think, be taken as an indication of a dramatic point of view, a mind capable of seeing both the imaginative and the practical aspects of thoughts and things ; the use to be made of which would depend on the powers and the tastes indicated elsewhere. It generally indicates also the gift of a humorous enjoyment of life and ideas.

A broken line is described by Desbarolles as

44

VI

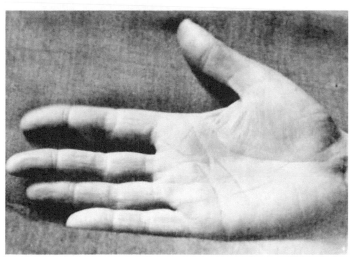

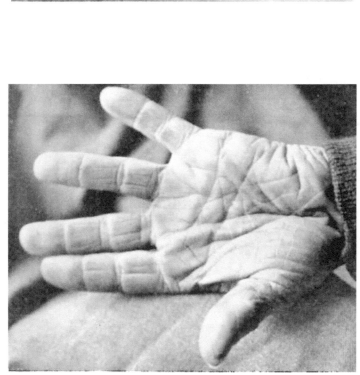

The Elementary type of hand. "Folds" rather than lines across the palm show that the intellectual capacities are in abeyance

The Idealistic type of hand. A strong Reason line shows constructive capacity and a branch to the Intuition line denotes insight and poise of mind

[face p. 44

foreboding death on the scaffold in a bad hand and signifying in a good hand a mortal head wound or the head being broken by accident. Herein he certainly mistakes, I think, effect for cause. It seems likely that a broken line would indicate a reason subject to eclipse; and this interpretation agrees with my own experience of such a line in hands I have been able frequently to observe. In a bad hand it would show the danger that moments of folly might occur, when reason could not restrain brutal action. In a good hand it would indicate rather a lapse of reason in a moment of danger, which might result in an accident. On the other hand, such moments of strain and danger might never occur in the lifetime of the individual. Desbarolles says he saw the broken line on the hands of two criminals who were hanged; but there certainly are more broken lines than executions and, in any case, no valid generalisation could be made from only two observations.

A broken line of Reason is therefore likely to mean that the mind, when agitated, would lose to a greater or lesser extent the power of Reason, or what is generally known as " presence of mind." Persons liable to such disturbance should avoid careers or occasions when dangerous

45

situations might demand instant decision. The truth of this interpretation of a broken line might easily be tested if a sufficient number of instances were taken ; and if confirmed would be a useful guide for education.

A wavy line that curves sometimes up and sometimes down indicates a Reason that inclines sometimes to emotional enjoyments of the instinctive life, sometimes more to the intellectual pleasures stimulated by intuitive feeling. Such a wavy line appears to be the sign of a vigorous mind and responsive nature ; but for intellectual work and development the instinctive emotions must be subordinated to the Reason and not deflect it from its path.

A very strong line dominating the whole palm, and seeming to have partly or wholly absorbed the higher line of Intuition, so that there are practically only two instead of three primary lines, is a formation I have referred to in a previous chapter as being often called " the murderer's line," but wrongly so as I think. It indicates a very powerful Reason which would dominate the mind and insist on such action as it decided was desirable in the circumstances, undeterred by instinctive fear or intuitive sympathy. It is obvious that such a line in a fine hand would not indicate the possibility of brutal deeds, though it might do so in the hand of an elementary or evilly-disposed person.

The line joined to the other two primary lines is described by Palmists as "a presage of misfortune"; and this is indeed likely to result from such a confusion of the capacities of Instinct, of Reason, and of Intuition. For a person whose right hand showed the joining of the lines, useful advice might be given as to some congenial pursuit that would induce the free development of Reason. Some course of study requiring concentrated thought would be best to advise. In this the mind might achieve a sense of power and well-being; and the growth of a branch to the line of Reason free from the entanglement would give tangible evidence of the improvement in the mind itself. I have actually seen such a branch develop in a hand that previously had the three lines deeply joined; and in this case, historical research coincided with the growth of a free branch to the line of Reason.

I have only twice seen the three lines joined together without any free branches, and this in both hands. These cases were those of imbecile children. It would be interesting to see what proportion of insane persons have such a formation of lines in their hands ; and this would be an investigation easy to carry out.

There is a formation sometimes called the Suicide line, which is mostly seen on the long thin hand known as that of the psychic type, where it would be more or less expected. I have not seen many hands of this type ; and when I have seen the line on hands of what is known as the mixed type, it has indicated what seems likely to be its meaning, as follows.

Such a line beginning very low down on the pad of imagination, sometimes sloping right up to the very centre of the base of the index finger, would indicate the imaginative Reason of a creative mind. This would be a very valuable asset for an artist, but dangerous for an undeveloped or ineffective mind, in which case its possessor might be tormented by un-coördinated images and become morbid. To use the Reason for some sort of constructive effort, no matter how humble, might relieve the over-burdened mind ; and advice to this effect in point of fact has been found useful.

A line beginning low but stopping short of the base of the index finger, or becoming merged in the line of Instinct, shows that the Reason would be of the imaginative kind, but without the power of expression shown by the upward ending.

The line of Reason deeply joined to the line of Instinct seems to show that one of the two faculties is subordinated to the other, and usually that the instinctive impulses govern the mind. With a strong line of Instinct, this is a quite usual formation in the hand of a man of action ; but for an individual desiring intellectual development, the instinctive impulses would need to be curbed. I have seen the two lines become separated where this discipline has been imposed. When both lines are weak, the person is likely to lack initiative and self-confidence.

A double line of Reason is seldom seen, and its meaning would depend on the relative position and strength of the two lines, as well as upon the other indications of the hand also. I can recall only three cases. Once, in the hands of a famous poet, I saw a second line above the ordinary one, and near to the line of Intuition. This seemed to me to indicate a faculty of Reason to function in transcendental as well as in practical spheres, but then I had already read the poet's verses. In another case, the second line was not nearly so strong ; and the rest of the hand showed that

E

there was more concern with material conditions and practical affairs. Still, the individual in question had poetical power and enjoyment of transcendental thought and feeling; and of this I was not aware at the time. In the third case, the line was strongly marked but occurred in a less cultured hand. I was somewhat at a loss for its meaning until my subject told me that she had lately developed the power of automatic writing. It was a chance meeting, and I have not seen the lady again; or I should have been interested to see the quality of what she wrote. The line is certainly not always present in the hands of those who practise automatic writing.

Spots or dents on the line I have always found a true indication of nervous overstrain or " brain fag," often causing headaches which are attributed to indigestion, chills and so on; whereas unless the brain is rested and refreshed, there will be no cure of the evil.

A line in " chains " shows that there are mental troubles, the cause of which may sometimes be deciphered in the upright lines. The indication is, as Desbarolles says, " a want of fixity of ideas, and sometimes migraine."

Islands on the line are said by the same author to indicate " prospects of murder, or shameful thoughts." " Cheiro " says they are " a sign of weakness from which, if they are strongly marked, the person will never recover." I have not been able to verify either of these drastic statements. It seems more likely that " islands " indicate some disorder of the brain that would temporarily affect the Reason. If this disorder could be foreseen, a warning of its approach might be very useful ; but I have no experience of the mark as foreboding a future state.

An entirely new position of the line may present a difficult problem for the Handreader. Considering its normal position as lying across the middle of the palm, midway between the lines of Instinct below and of Intuition above, any deviation to a higher or lower position of the line of Reason may, roughly speaking, be construed as indicating a mind absorbed either in the material affairs of life or the emotional feelings and desires if it is set low. If running high and near the base of the fingers, intellectual interests or idealistic feelings are indicated.

A line connecting the two upper primary lines, Plate VI, is said by " Cheiro " to " foreshadow some great fascination or affection at which moment the subject will be blind to reason and danger." I think that the sudden realisation of a great love is only one form in which the power indicated by the line might function. Individuals who have what we may regard as a pathway along which messages from the Intuition can travel to the Reason, would be able to obtain a quick perception of the truth and import of many different situations and affairs. In an elementary hand the line might indicate a grasp of quite simple and practical matters ; in a finer hand the understanding might be that of intellectual truth. In both cases the individual would feel that his mind was inspired at times beyond its normal perceptive power. In the very rare cases in which I have seen such a line in hands of a fine shape, the individuals undoubtedly possessed a unique poise of mind, felt by other people as a superior quality which could not be exactly analysed, but which diffused a sense of harmonious well-being and happiness to those in contact with them.

CHAPTER V

THE third primary line, which Palmists call the *Heart Line*, I renamed the line of *Intuition*, because I found the meaning of "heart" so unsuitable to the significance of the line, as marked in the hands of people who had unusual ones. I found that individuals who had this line strongly marked and in a good position high in the palm had sensitive minds of an intellectual or idealistic nature. They invariably had also the gift of intuition, used either for expression in art or thought, or for the affairs of life. The only "heart" affairs marked on the line by *breaks, chains, islands,* etc., were those that caused sorrow, great disappointment, or remorse; and these would naturally affect the intuitive capacity. All the sex affairs and influences of other people that affect the life are marked either on the instinctive or imaginative portion of the hand. This third and highest primary line is likely to show rather the powers of intellectual sympathy and insight; and this I have always found to be the case. Possibly *heart* bears a different significance in these days than when it was first adopted in Palmistry. In Pascal's oft-quoted " The heart hath its reasons which the reason doth not know," the word *heart* is used almost in the sense in which I use the word Intuition, as meaning an intellectual perception rather than an instinctive feeling. The expressions, " warm-hearted," " heart affairs," etc., place the word *heart* in a different category. Reading, in his *Introduction to Metaphysics*, Bergson's definition of Intuition as " a kind of intellectual sympathy " decided my adoption of the name Intuition instead of Heart for the third primary line.

A strong, clear line beginning high in the cleft between the index and middle finger (Plate VI) indicates a power of true and sympathetic feeling; the nearer to the index finger, the more it shows the idealistic quality.

A good line beginning in the very centre of the base of the index finger (Plate VIII) indicates in the hand of an artist or man of thought a gift of creative insight. In a practical hand such a line would show the power of the mind to go " to the very heart of the matter "—or person—dealt

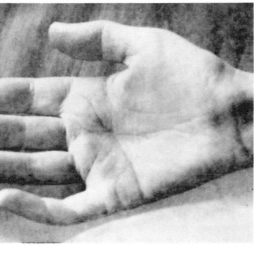

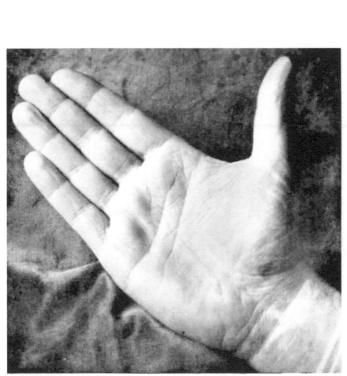

Strong Intuition line turning *down* to Instinct shows intuitive capacity for business. The greater width across the base of the hand denotes practical enterprise. The "spear head" on base of index finger implies political ability

Strong Intuition line here turns *upwards*, denoting the artistic creative insight. The narrow base of the hand and flatness of the ball of the thumb shows weak instinctive dispositions. The width across the base of fingers shows enterprise in Art

LINE OF INTUITION OR " HEART LINE "

with. It is the power of gaining an intimate knowledge of men and things that cannot as a rule be fully grasped by the reason, but is felt to be a sure and certain apprehension of the truth.

A strong line beginning on the border of the hand below the base of the index finger indicates the intuitive faculty of a teacher or ruler, and a creative power over other minds.

A strong line dipping down to the line of Instinct (Plate VII) shows that the intuitive faculty is used for the affairs of life, business, politics, etc. The way it is, or should be, used may be learnt from the comparative strength of the fingers and their bases, the lines of Instinct and Imagination, and the upright or secondary lines.

A line beginning low under the middle finger shows that the intuitive faculty is not strong. Sympathy and Insight would not then guide the mind, but if either the Reason or the Instinct is good, it would be the ruling power. Where all three lines are weak and there is no outstanding power indicated, life is likely to be ordinary though not necessarily unhappy or useless. On the contrary, people of such natures, being well-balanced, are often more easily contented—that is if all the other dispositions are normal—and can make a happy atmosphere around them that is helpful to more energetic minds. Luckily, such individuals are not rare; for if everyone were a genius or a crank the world would not be a pleasant place to live in. Well-balanced and harmonious natures are very valuable, if they do not allow themselves to become cabbages. Handreaders will find such hands less exciting than the abnormal ones, but for study they provide material for good practice since in them the student must look for slight differences.

High up in the hand the line indicates that the intuitive faculty is more concerned with idealistic than practical affairs; set low that it is used more for practical interests.

Breaks in the line indicate some shock to the sensitiveness of the mind, not only arising from love affairs, but also from sorrows, shocks, or other causes.

Red patches on the line seem to indicate that the intuition is being overwrought, or blinded by passion. I have seen this condition of the line when the mind was clouded by acute jealousy; and this may be the reason why the line has been called that of the " heart "; but Desbarolles says that in the hands of criminals, and especially of parricides, the line is the colour of blood. A mind pervaded by passion would lose the power of intellectual insight; and the line indicating the faculty of Intuition would show breaks and blotches in consequence.

The entire absence of the line would indicate that the mind lacked the capacity of Intuition. In most cases this would be a serious drawback to other powers. When, however, the line is simply absorbed by the line of Reason, it might, in a good hand, indicate something in the nature of genius. The two faculties could, so to speak, work together; but this meaning would only apply where the two lines were obviously merged in one. Where the line is entirely absent, the want of intellectual sympathy must be reckoned with.

When I have seen the lines of Reason and Intuition linked together by branches or by definite lines such as the marking called " the mystic cross," I have always found that the individual had, in some degree, that special gift of understanding which springs from some movement within the mind itself and does not depend on any stimulus or sensory perception.

CHAPTER VI

THE THUMB

THE thumb is a very important member of the hand ; and it gives indications of the possession or absence of very important qualities of mind. The truth of the association of these qualities with the shape of the thumb can easily be ascertained ; for the set and size of the thumbs of many individuals whose qualities are known can be observed without difficulty.

The thumb represents something in the nature of " an idea of the self " in the mind. Individuals with big thumbs are generally dominating and assertive of their own purpose and will. Individuals with short thumbs are not as a rule self-assertive or strong willed, though they may be obstinate if the thumb is thick.

A large thumb set low on the hand and lying at right angles to it when the hand is open, indicates a strong and independent disposition somewhat apt to go to extremes. A small thumb in this position indicates merely an impulsive disposition.

A thumb set high on the hand and inclining

towards the fingers indicates a reserved and, if exaggerated, an over-cautious disposition.

Adaptability is the quality shown by an outward bend of the nail joint of the thumb. Generosity or extravagance are often said to be indicated by this. I think that these qualities spring from the adaptability of the individual to a given situation or to the needs of others ; and danger of extravagance arises only when the judgment is weak or the mind deranged.

A stiff joint is indicative of a reserved or egoistic nature and a non-adaptable personality. This would be a good formation for the thumb of a gifted artist, but dangerous for an undeveloped mind. In the latter case adaptability to the opinions and needs of others would be a more valuable quality.

A thumb that turned inwards, unless the other indications of the hand were fine, would indicate a lack of responsiveness that might induce meanness.

A thumb with a very strong outward bend would indicate a nature apt to be too responsive ; and the subject should be advised to cultivate restraint and the delay of action till judgment has time to direct it. Quick sympathy can hardly be controlled ; but a habit of restraint can be established in a child's education. To learn to restrain one's own mind is perhaps a more difficult matter.

The individual's power of Will and Judgment is indicated by the two phalanges or joints of the thumb.

The nature, and sometimes even the existence, of the Will is disputed, but most people agree there is a particular quality or power possessed by some individuals that is generally called a strong will. For our present purposes this may be defined as a power of sustaining opinions or efforts till the desired end is achieved. It is a kind of mental energy. The strength of this in the individual is indicated by the thickness and length of the nail or second joint of the thumb.

The nail joint long and also thick indicates a fine and strong will, which will give the strength of purpose necessary for the full development and use of the mental powers and tastes of the individual.

A long thin nail joint is appropriate to the thumb of an abstract thinker, which might not need determination for practical purposes. A somewhat short, thick joint is more suitable in the thumb of a manual worker, as it shows the determination necessary for practical rather than for intellectual interests.

THE THUMB

I have never seen a nail joint of the thumb that seemed too long. It would indicate a despotic will, the use of which would depend on the instincts, talents, tastes, and desires, which are shown by the other lines and parts of the hand.

The nail joint both short and thin signifies a weak will; and in this case any qualities or tastes otherwise indicated must be largely discounted.

If the nail joint of a child's thumb indicated a weakness of will and his behaviour also showed a lack of purpose, it would be all the more important to concentrate on the development of any special interests and tastes shown by the rest of the hand. Wise guidance could establish these as habits, whereas otherwise they might degenerate, and the mind become discontented or futile owing to want of interests which the unaided will was too weak to develop.

A splayed out tip to the thumb is said by Desbarolles to be a very bad sign, indicating violent temper and brutal or murderous acts. The only time I have seen such a thumb was on the hand of a mild-looking grocer's assistant. I regarded him well for some time but could see no other indication of brutality and I lacked the courage to question him as to his hidden feelings and propensities.

The first phalange or joint of the thumb (sometimes called the second) is significant of the individual's power of instinctive or impulsive judgment. This differs from the power of intellectual judgment which is shown by the middle primary line in the palm. Judgments or opinions of the sort indicated by the thumb are quickly made and do not need reflection. The individual who makes them is said " to know his own mind " ; but he may not be able to give the reason for his opinions.

A long thick joint indicates the possession of a good judgment or " common sense " ; if very thick there is an inclination to be obstinate.

Long and thin, the joint points to a fine power of discrimination ; and if it is " waisted " it means a tactful nature.

When short and thick this joint shows an obstinate and, if the Reason is poor, a stupid nature. If the line of Reason is good, however, the individual would simply be " slow in making up his mind."

A very small joint compared with the rest of the hand, or one that is badly shaped, shows a poor instinctive judgment. Where the line of Reason is good, this may not greatly matter ; but Reason is a slow, deliberate process, more useful to a man of thought than to a man of action.

THE THUMB

The ball of the thumb is not a third phalange but part of the hand, and the pad on it is scientifically known as " the thenar eminence." It is enclosed by the primary line of Instinct and seems to be correlated with the part of the brain that deals with mental processes concerned with instinct, the emotions, and impulsive actions. Roughly speaking, it indicates instinctive reactions to sensory stimuli, and the instinctive dispositions, desires and cravings of the nature.

The sex instinct is evidently of great importance ; but to call the ball of the thumb " the mount of Venus " seems to ascribe too large a part of the instinctive life to sex feelings and impulses. The nature, scope and classification of the instincts is much disputed by modern psychologists ; but we may define an instinct for our present purposes as any disposition to feel and act spontaneously in certain definite ways without reflection or reasoned decision— often, indeed, in spite of them. The behaviour which issues from the instinctive dispositions shows purposefulness, for it is generally serviceable to the creature, or its kind, and looks as if it were guided by intelligence.

When the base of the thumb is very large and full compared with the rest of the hand, it indicates strong instinctive dispositions, the power of enjoyment, the love of beauty in nature and in art, especially music—in short a pleasure-loving nature.

A full and soft pad indicates a nature that cares for sensuous enjoyments rather than practical activities ; and, if the fullness is mostly on the middle of the pad, sex is likely to play a large part in the person's life. When such fullness is observed on the outer side, it shows an affectionate and sociable or philanthropic nature, rather than an emphasis on sex. When it is mostly on the part just under the index finger, it denotes a strong combative instinct. The subject displaying fullness here would be likely to be " up against " people and usually accepted ideas. This is a dangerous attitude to life ; but it can be countered by a habit of calm reflection and the cultivation of a sense of humour. To be able to hold your own, however, is very useful in important matters.

A hard thin pad indicates a nature not greatly concerned with love or sex or the enjoyment of sensuous pleasures.

Hard and full, it is a sign of a love of practical, energetic and emotional interests rather than of pleasures.

64

A square on the pad is said to indicate danger of imprisonment or detention in a hospital, and I have seen it and interpreted it correctly as an indication of the latter.

The ball of the thumb is often covered with fine lines which show, I think, unsatisfied desires, and a restless, impulsive mind. When there are only a few fine lines here, the nature finds interest in serious pursuits or is a cold and indifferent one.

I have not paid attention to the lines on the ball of the thumb unless they cross the line of Instinct. When this happens, their significance is to be noted by the point at which they touch or cross other lines, which will be dealt with later on.

I understand that some professional Palmists pay great attention to this part of the hand, and " Cheiro " says the Hindus and Gipsies base their calculations largely on it. I fancy the concentration of a Palmist's attention on this portion of the hand, which is, we assume, corre-lated with the instinctive part of one's mental make up, would be most favourable for the reception of telepathic impressions. In any case, further consideration of the lines and marks on the ball of the thumb would be interesting.

CHAPTER VII

THE index finger is the finger of authority. How often in our childhood an upright index finger has emphasized a warning to us or, held straight out, pointed a direction with authoritative, and almost hypnotic power.

This finger was aptly named after Jupiter, the chief of the Roman gods ; for it represents the aspirations and ambitions of the intellect and is certainly a most powerful member of the hand, though the thumb may perhaps be the most useful. These two are the only fingers that normally can be held erect apart from the others.

The mound at the base of the finger is important ; it seems to be correlated with the initiation of new thoughts and efforts (mental creativeness) and a desire for personal supremacy. I have more often seen new lines appear on this mound than on any other part of the hand. Generally these new lines are branches from the lines of Reason and Intuition, which I think indicates that either the thoughts or feelings of the mind are striving for expression in some definite form. The length and proportions of the finger itself would give one some idea of the direction in which the striving proceeds. Strangely enough, these lines have often appeared before the individuals possessing them were aware that their minds were stretching out towards some definite achievement ; but when the lines and their meaning have been pointed out, they realised for the first time this new push of their natures. I feel that this realisation is of value, and have accordingly given special attention to the meaning of lines and marks on the base of the index finger.

A long, powerful index finger with a full base in a good well-shaped hand, indicates a leader or an initiator in thought or action. If the nail phalange is the most developed, the leadership will be possibly in ethics or some ideal thought. Should the middle phalange dominate, the person might excel in science or art. The first phalange (next the hand) indicates initiation or leadership in practical affairs.

A strong finger with a flat base shows a proud and ambitious nature with power for action rather than for ideas ; but the primary lines and the thumb must always be considered in determining the direction which the ambition would take.

A long thin finger indicates a mind interested in new ideas, though without the power or ambition to influence others.

A short finger with a flat base points to a lack of ambition or of interest in creative ideas. With a full base it shows a mind that enjoys new ideas of other people ; and in a practical hand it goes with a love of Nature and outdoor life.

A stumpy finger means pride without ambition ; and with a flat base it means a lack of interest in ideas.

The most usual length for the finger nowadays is slightly shorter than the ring finger. Dr. Vaschide says " le canon de la beauté parfaite des mains " is for the index finger to be longer than the ring finger (this is shown in Plate II, the most beautiful hand I have seen, also in Plate VI) ; but in an examination of the hands of a hundred French women he found that only ten per cent. had the index finger longer than, and six per cent. of equal length with, the ring finger. Men had an even less proportion, and my experience coincides with his. In old pictures of beautiful women I have noticed that the hand is always painted with a long index finger, which certainly gives it an elegant appearance; but I think we may consider an almost equal length of the two fingers as normal and a much longer or shorter index finger as significant.

Desbarolles insists that a cross attached to a star on the base of the index finger indicates an important marriage, because he has so frequently seen these marks on the hands of women who had married grandees or very rich men. It seems more likely that these marks indicate something in the nature of mental activity in the initiation of new ideas or ambitious projects. In the case of some women, these can only be fulfilled by a prosperous marriage; but this would only be a means to their end of aggrandisement. A woman who had intellectual or artistic gifts could attain power through her talents, and would be likely to have the same mark; which I think promises success because it indicates a strength of purpose to achieve expression for a dominating personality. The wives of many famous men have no such mark in their hands. I remember to have seen it only in one case; and then it seemed to show the ambition of the nature rather than the marriage.

A cross alone Desbarolles says indicates " a love marriage, often a happy one."

A star alone is a sign of unexpected honours and satisfied ambition, according to the same author.

A triangle means success in diplomatic organisation, arrangement or invention. This I have frequently seen as a sign that the mind had an unusual gift for successful organisation of social or commercial affairs.

A square points to preservation from the danger of overweening pride and ambition.

A spear head indicates political ambition and aptitude; and this curious mark is clearly visible in the print of Gladstone's hand given in "Cheiro's" book. I saw a similar mark on the hands of a clever young man, Plate VIII, of whose political ambitions I was unaware before I had read his hands.

A trident in the centre of the base of the finger indicates that great success will be won through the magnetic power of the personality over other people. Only once have I seen the Trident clearly and perfectly formed. The owner of this rare mark was a famous man; and his friends told me they had never before heard his peculiar quality so well described. A Trident not perfectly formed would still indicate magnetic power in a lesser degree ; and this I have several times found a true indication. The power itself is unmistakable though it is difficult to analyse.

CHAPTER VIII

THE OTHER FINGERS

THE middle finger, the ring finger, and the little finger, called respectively Saturn, Apollo and Mercury in the old systems, give indications of the inherited dispositions and tastes of the mind.

If the hand is held out with the fingers fully extended, their comparative length and size can be easily noted. A wide space between the index and middle fingers is said to show independence of thought, or between the ring and little fingers, independence of action. I am not sure that these indications can be relied on, but when the trend of the mind is otherwise doubtfully shown, they may be useful supplements to other indications.

A strong middle finger indicates in a good hand a religious or studious disposition. In a weak hand these might degenerate into superstition or morbidness.

A small middle finger would show a lack of interest in deep or serious subjects, and in a weak hand stupidity.

A crooked middle finger indicates an evil disposition or imbecility.

A strong ring finger (Plates VIII and IX), long and well proportioned, in a good hand indicates a joyous disposition, a love of beauty in art and life, and, together with a full base, a power of artistic expression ; but if the hand is weak and the indications of intellect poor, the disposition may be of a frivolous nature. A thick first phalange—next the hand—indicates a love of sensuous beauty ; the second one shows a love of nature or science. The nail phalange, if strong, shows a love of abstract or ideal beauty ; and generally, with a full base, it is a mark of the disposition of a poet or painter.

A long thin finger is said to show a love of society and frequently a gambling disposition ; but I have not verified this.

When the base of the ring finger is full just under the finger itself, it indicates a love of colour and harmony in art ; if however it inclines towards the middle finger it shows more studious tastes. In the cleft towards the little finger, a practical use of the sense of colour and harmony in the affairs of life is indicated.

An important little finger (called Mercury) (Plate VII), indicates generally a man of affairs, such as finance, politics or business. When very long it is said to indicate an orator ; and a print of Gladstone's hand shows the little finger nearly as long as the ring finger. I have always found a power of speaking well in public associated with a little finger even slightly longer than usual, but so far I have not seen the hand of a potential Gladstone.

The base of the little finger gives some idea of the organising power of the individual. When large, full and square-set to the finger, a strong and practical businesslike ability is indicated. Sloping down, towards the outer border of the hand, the power of organising would be for social affairs, to do with people rather than with business.

Two deep, perpendicular lines on the base of the little finger are said to indicate " a good Doctor or a good Nurse." Clever doctors sometimes have these lines and sometimes do not. I have more often seen them on the hands of good nurses. I do not remember seeing them except on the hands of those engaged in some form of medical or social work.

The first phalange of the little finger when long and thick shows ability for commerce ; the second

74

X

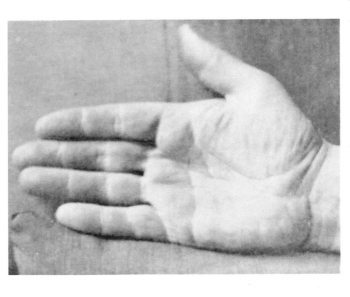

The same hand a year later, showing the growth of creative power by development of the base of index finger. The line of Personality also shows improvement and success

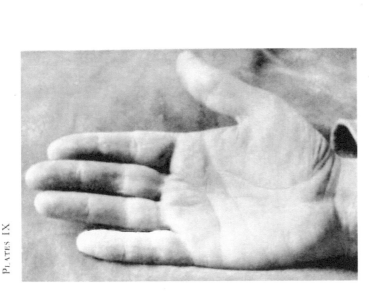

A painter's talent is shown by powerful ring finger. The full base of the hand indicates great imaginative and emotional power

phalange points to scientific tastes ; and the nail phalange, if unusually long and thick, indicates inventive ability, the value and success of which will depend on the other powers of the mind.

CHAPTER IX

IMAGINATION

THE imaginative powers of the mind seem to be correlated with the ulnar border of the hand, or the portion termed by anatomists the hypothenar eminence, which extends from the wrist to the base of the little finger. Palmists call it the " Mount of Luna " ; but since they all agree that it represents the imagination, let us discard the term " Luna," as well as " hypothenar," and speak of the eminence of Imagination.

A full, firm eminence indicates that the imagination is strong and active, and that it forms a good counterpart to the instinctive tendencies shown by a good base of the thumb. This balance is most important. The whole base of the hand, as we have seen, is composed of the two portions that represent for us Instinct and Imagination. Both are needed in right proportions as a basis for the full development of the mental capacities.

A human being without Imagination might not attain to full intellectual power, though possibly he might be "intelligent" and purposeful by reason of his instinctive energy. Without the driving power of instinct, the Imagination lacks force and incentive. Accordingly, when indications of a fine Imagination are observed, look also to see whether it is well balanced by a good Instinct.

The part near the wrist may be termed primitive Imagination. If strong and full and square-set to the wrist, it denotes perseverance ; but if flat and sloping away towards the wrist it shows a lack of that quality. The mind is apparently unable to hold the image of the desired act long enough for it to be carried out without difficulty.

The middle portion of the eminence indicates reflective or constructive Imagination, which is important in connection with a good line of Reason. Great fullness in this portion, when it is almost a cushion of soft tissue, denotes strong moods which give great power to constructive ideas. To a certain degree, moodiness can replace perseverance when this is lacking. When in the mood the individual can do great things ; but power goes when the mood changes, for the idea supporting and nourishing it has faded.

The part of the eminence just under the line of Intuition Palmists call the "Mount of Mars." I think it represents rather the power of Imagination to give courage and self-control to the mind, both in physical and mental difficulties, so that an ideal of conduct can be firmly held in such a way as to dominate instinctive impulses and fears. I have always found this portion of the eminence, when both full and firm, to be associated with the power of self-control. " Cheiro " also considers that it indicates " Passive courage, resignation and strength of resistance against wrong " ; but to my mind these are included under the meaning of self-control, which, as we have said, is induced by the power of a fine imagination.

A full but soft and flabby eminence indicates a sensuous Imagination which would be a danger except in a person of strong intellect.

A thin, hard eminence shows a poor Imagination. In a very fine hand this might be compensated by an unusually good line of Intuition.

A heavy line across the lower part of the eminence, I conclude, is an indication of something in the nature of an inherited scar or obsession of the mind for drink or drugs. There is always a danger for persons exhibiting such a line that the temptation will crop up in the life of the individual ; but from what I have been often told, this may be of the nature of a passing thought only and always seems alien to the personality even if indulged in for a time.

Lines across what is called the percussion or outside edge of the hand that come on to the eminence, are said to indicate voyages. I think a change, or a new point of view, is a better description of their meaning. This is, of course, frequently coincident with a voyage, but may equally well be the result of reading a clever book, or meeting a striking personality, or any other mental stimulus. The more of these the better if they stir the imagination to new ideas and activities.

CHAPTER X

THE shape of the hand does not show to what profession or occupation the individual belongs, but indicates the inherited dispositions and general tendency of the mind to be elementary, or practical, or enterprising, or studious, or artistic, or sensitive, or a blend of all six, which it usually is.

Palmists generally ascribe so many meanings to each of the different shapes of the hand that the result is extremely confusing. The whole nature and power of the mind cannot be gathered from the shape alone. Indeed this is often misleading as to the intellectual capacities; for, if the indications of these are unusually good, they can override the limitations of the inherited dispositions.

Hands are divided into seven types by D'Arpentigny, as follows :—

    I.   The elementary, or lowest type of hand (Plate V).

II.   The square, or useful hand (Plate XII).
III. The spatulate, or active type (Plate IV).
IV. The knotty, or philosophic hand.
V.   The conic, or artistic type (Plate XI).
VI. The psychic, or idealistic hand (Plate VI).
VII. The mixed hand.

I have never seen hands that belonged entirely to any one type except the mixed. One finger may be conic, another spatulate, and so on. However, the hand, as a whole, generally shows a predominating tendency towards one " pure " type or another.

Unless there is some unusual feature or some problem of the mind to be solved, I do not think it is necessary greatly to consider the shape of the hand. It is, however, important to remember that strong, clear, upright lines are less significant in long, thin hands of the psychic or the artistic type than in square or spatulate hands. The psychic type especially has very deep, upright lines as a rule. I think the term " psychic " is not well suited to the long, thin hand, for the word is associated with Spiritualism and occult interests, whereas the particular tendencies associated with hands of this type are those of an inquiring and sensitive mind, useful for any pursuit or professsion for which the individual is otherwise fitted. Lawyers, scientists, doctors —even pickpockets—may all have "psychic hands," but it is unusual for artists to have this shape ; though, indeed, art seems to have a greater variety of minds engaged in her service than there are in any other profession. The genius of artists is shown more by the lines than by the shape of their hands, which are sometimes conic, or square, or spatulate, and sometimes even of the knotty type.

A spatulate palm is a helpful indication of an enterprising mind. If the spatulate part (or greater width) is at the base of the hand (Plates IV and VII), the individual is likely to be enterprising in the active and practical affairs of life or business. If the greater width is across the base of the fingers (Plate VIII), enterprise would more likely be in art or intellectual interests.

Spatulate finger tips also indicate an enterprising disposition and an original way of regarding things. I think it far better to allot only those two meanings to the spread-out of the finger tips, and let the other parts of the hand yield each its own significance. The disposition to regard everything in an original way, indicated by the spatulate finger tips, could be used in any avocation for which the individual was fitted, but it would not indicate his particular way of life, or vocation.

Very square finger tips with broad nails show a critical disposition.

Square finger tips with long or almond-shaped nails indicate a sensible, good-tempered disposition.

Conic or rounded finger tips show an artistic or pleasure-loving disposition.

Pointed finger tips refer to a refined and, if long, to an idealistic disposition. If they are very short it is an indication of frivolity.

Flexible fingers show an impressionable disposition and, if very flexible— almost to the point of being double-jointed— the indication is that of a mind so easily dominated by the impression of the moment that it is unstable. However, if the will is developed and strong enough to resist the over-dominance of the feeling of the moment (and this can generally be effected) the impressionable personality can also be a very charming one.

Stiff fingers indicate a reserved, sometimes even a hard or cruel disposition. Individuals with stiff fingers cannot respond easily to the feeling of the moment ; though an otherwise good hand might show fine qualities, reserve would be likely to hide them. Gracious manners should certainly be cultivated by such people in order to do themselves justice. Modification of an over-reserved and also too impressionable nature can certainly be effected by the average individual who has inherited and not formed these dispositions ; but such discipline should be begun early in life, although practicable at any time.

Naturally crooked fingers (not due to rheumatism) on a bad or weak hand are said to point to evil dispositions and, on a good hand, to quizzical and irritating tendencies.

I have often found a crooked little finger a sign of contrariness, sometimes even perversity. To be aware that this little demon of a tendency is part of their inherited nature helps individuals first to recognise, then to laugh at, and finally to suppress the malign efforts of the imp to frustrate not only other people's wishes but even their own desires.

The nails provide very clear evidence of the state of the nerves and could often give a useful warning that they are being over-tried and need rest and refreshment. It is so easy to say " don't worry " ; but if the skin round the nails is breaking or splitting it is usually due to over-fussing, and this is as detrimental to the mind as it is to the nails. Unless matters are improved and peace is restored to the mind, the nails themselves will in time show splits and break easily at the edges. This means a really serious overstrain or weakness, and medical consultation would be advisable.

From what I have seen, read, and heard of the diagnosis of disease from the shape of the hand and the nails, I feel confident that it is a great mistake to attempt it. Doctors already have far more accurate sources of information at their disposal and, I believe, know the indications given by the nails, which they find helpful in some cases. In the present state of our knowledge all matters relating to organic diseases and to health are best left to medical men. Let Handreaders concentrate on the analysis of the mental characteristics, and the possibility of the moral and intellectual development of the personality. This may assist the physical health also, for the power and purpose of the mind when aroused to full activity infuses a sense of well-being throughout the whole organism.

Temperament is indicated by the formation and cushions of the palm. I give in parallel columns the descriptions and their indications.

Description.	*Indication.*
A firm and well covered palm.	A quick, cheerful temperament.
A soft and well covered palm.	An indolent temperament.
A very soft and very thick palm.	A sensual temperament.
A hard, well covered palm.	An energetic temperament.
A thin and hard palm.	A cold and restless temperament.
A thin and soft palm.	A lethargic temperament.
Criss-crossed with fine lines.	An irritable or worrying temperament.

A hollow palm is said to indicate misfortune, and this seems to be true. The lack of joyous experience may affect the bodily tissue and cause " hollowness " ; though this may seem a far-fetched explanation.

Temperament is often blamed for excesses of all sorts ; and, if a person is judged by the signs to be very " temperamental," the Handreader must consider it as a possible hindrance to the success of the ambitions. Unless the palm, however, is very unusually thick, or soft, or hard, it really needs only a passing glance.

" Cheiro " affirms that large hands generally do very fine work and love great detail. Small hands, on the contrary, prefer to carry out large ideas and dislike detail. I have not given enough attention to the shape of hands to have an opinion as to the truth of this statement, nor have I read

D'Arpentigny's book on the subject. Now that photography makes a large collection of hand-prints possible for comparison and analysis, the study of the shape and markings of hands on a sufficiently scientific wide scale might be undertaken with great advantage. The truth and value of Palmistry could thus be thoroughly tested.

CHAPTER XI

THE fascination of deciphering the plan of the future is attached to the secondary or upright lines in the palm. This is not fortune telling. Though otherwise inaccessible to observation, the purposeful pattern of the organism, or the dream of the mind for the fruition of its powers, seems to be unfolded in the upright lines of the hand. As it is improbable that all the chances of life which must be encountered can be foreseen, the future of the individual cannot be confidently predicted. Yet a strong personality is not easily frustrated by circumstance. A good thumb and clear, strong, upright lines betoken a firmness of purpose which, in spite of all obstacles, may fulfil the vision of the mind.

Of the two principal upright lines, Palmists call one that of " Fate " and the other that of " Apollo," or Fortune, or the line of the Sun. This latter line I have renamed " Personality " ;

Plate XI

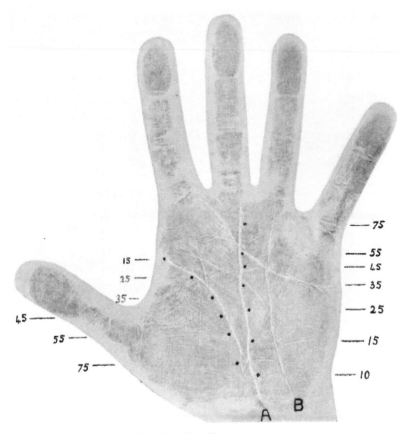

A. The Fate line
B. The line of Personality

Points give approximate dates. The age runs *down* the Instinct line and *up* the Fate line

as it clearly seems to portray the development of the inner self or ego and its expression in art or life. The Fate line I called for some time the line of " Environment," which better describes its significance; but Environment is a tiresome word and in any case *is* Fate unless conquered by the personality. I have accordingly reverted to the use of the term Fate for the central upright line.

In the beginning of my study I was puzzled by the inappropriateness of the meanings assigned by Desbarolles and also by " Cheiro " to a strong line of Fate, and also by the significance they attached to the absence of the line. My own experience so often showed both meanings to be entirely wrong. A strong line of Fate, they aver, going unbroken from the wrist to the base of the middle finger, indicates " extreme good fortune and success." Now I frequently found such lines in the hands of poor and unfortunate people. It is true that I also saw such lines in the hands of rich people, but they were not always happy. On the contrary, they were often discontented or bored with life, and one cannot call that " great good fortune and success."

Moreover, the absence of the line, Desbarolles says, is the sign of an insignificant existence. I have found, on the contrary, that highly gifted persons with successful careers exhibited little or no line of Fate. In their case it was often entirely supplanted by the line of Personality, which then ruled the palm as the chief line.

My own conclusions are that we may regard the line of Fate as representing the outer circumstances of life which have either been inherited or provided by others. If these are agreeable they may absorb all the interest and energy of the mind ; while if unsatisfactory they may cause hardship or discontent. In any case, they represent Fate and they can only be changed by such an effort of the personality to assert its own independence that environment will cease to dominate the life or to dictate its interests. Probably the fashionable folk who visited Desbarolles and " Cheiro " were mostly people well satisfied with the inherited positions and riches indicated by their strong lines of Fate, and so misled the Palmists as to the bed-rock meaning of the line. Little or no line of Fate means, I think, that the mind and life are open to other influences than those forced on individuals by inherited circumstances. Without personal gifts or powers of any sort (which is unusual) there might not be what is understood by success. But life is generally interesting, and the Hand-reader need not regret the absence of the line.

The line of Fate usually commences from or near to the wrist, and is strongest in the early portion when the child is entirely compassed by the home influences. If the line persists strong and unbroken this early influence of the environment continues ; and, unless there is a still stronger line of Personality, the mental life is restricted by material conditions. These may be either those of great riches or those of great poverty, and who shall say which is the most formidable obstacle to the growth of a free personality ?

A strong line of Fate going unbroken right up to the middle finger (Plate XI) would indicate that worldly cares or family ties are likely to be the chief concern of the mind throughout life. This does not, of course, by any means preclude happiness, or misery, or the enjoyment of intellectual and artistic pursuits ; but it does indicate that the latter will be subordinated to what is well expressed as " life."

A line stopping below the line of Reason indicates the breaking away from early environment.

Usually in such a case a new line then begins, which indicates rather the individual's own choice, and if the new line begins before the other leaves off, the change is one towards better conditions.

A new line that comes from Imagination, and either supplants or closely accompanies the line of Fate (Plate III), generally indicates a happy and prosperous marriage. It may mean a friendship or companionship only, but it is always a sign of a good and helpful influence in one's life. I have very frequently seen this line in the hands of girls who afterwards made happy marriages, which I conclude were largely brought about by the imaginative wish of their minds, marriage being, as it were, their vocation.

Lines that approach from the line of Imagination but do not break or continue alongside the Fate line, indicate engagements or influences that do not continue. A line that breaks the Fate line and then stops abruptly, seems to indicate some misfortune to the love affair, or a shock caused by death or accident.

Lines crossing the Fate line, running across that of Instinct from the base of the thumb (Plate III), show the sex desires and influences that affect one's life. They are seldom good or helpful indications, as they more often cross the line with a downward slope. This appears to be always a sign of adverse influence; but, if the line turns upwards after crossing the line of Fate, and runs towards the little finger, it may indicate a happy marriage, the foundation of which will be that of an instinctive urge, or sensuous love, rather than the more ideal love shown if the line should originate from the eminence of Imagination.

Continuations of the Fate line are, I think, better named lines of Initiative (Plate IV). They are lines springing from the line of Instinct, and if strong, always indicate a new and successful achievement on the part of the individual, won by his personal merit; and this is distinctly *not* due to Fate or the influence of others. I have often seen such lines correctly indicating the time when the individual launched out on his own. Even if the central Fate line continues as the strongest line, and there is only a thin thread of the line of *Initiative*, it indicates that there has been, or will be, a strong instinctive urge to some enterprise, of the nature and origin of which the individual is often not fully conscious. These lines seem to represent the striving of the whole instinctive nature to express its purpose and power through conscious action.

The line of Initiative tending towards the Index Finger, in an artistic hand, would indicate new creative freedom and power. In a practical hand, it would mean successful ambition in the pursuit engaged in. If the line goes towards any of the other fingers, success would be won in the interests they represent.

Breaks in the line of Fate indicate changes in the environment and are nearly always good, more especially if a good line begins before the old one leaves off. A line made up of a number of little breaks shows a continuous change for the better, what Desbarolles describes as " une échelle pour monter."

Islands on the line always point to trouble of some sort, though Desbarolles says they may indicate " bonheur par l'adultère." " Cheiro " thinks islands are marks of misfortune, loss or adversity. My own experience suggests that the environment is, so to speak, " split " either by love or disgrace, or both. The island expresses this dividing of the mental life between different interests, or two streams of conscious contact with circumstances. I have often seen these curious " islands " as true indications of some trouble in the past; but I have not seen them as coming in the future. The lines that form them sometimes fade when the time of stress is over, and sometimes remain for many years. I have never seen one that was not a true mark of past trouble of some sort at the date indicated.

Squares on the line are said to be marks of preservation from danger of some sort. I am still greatly puzzled by these " squares "; they have been so invariably true as signs that the mind has received some sudden illumination or help in dangers of various sorts. Those occurring on or near the line of Fate have in my experience meant that anxieties caused by moral difficulties, or financial losses, have been unexpectedly removed. Sometimes at the last moment a way out has been revealed.

Crosses on the line I have never seen; but the meaning of little lines that cross it depends on the place from which they come and where they end. Coming from the line of Instinct and just touching the line of Fate, they are generally indications of interference in material affairs, usually caused by relations. Such lines show that one's life is too easily affected by impulsive thoughts and feelings. It is extremely hard for some natures to curb these; but I have been told that being made aware that one would gain happiness by the effort to do so has helped to good results, and life has become less fretted by the interference of other people.

CHAPTER XII

THE LINE OF PERSONALITY

THIS line has been called that of Apollo, the line of Fortune, and sometimes the Sun line; but none of these names helps to elucidate or express its meaning. It seems to represent the personal ideas or the spirit of the individual; and this inner power of the mind is best conveyed, I think, by the word Personality.

A strong line dominating the palm indicates the success of the imaginative self and desires, whether for artistic expression or for love, or fame, or riches, or power. A poor artist in a garret who had succeeded in expressing his art to his own satisfaction, might well have this strong line of Personality, while it might be absent from the hand of a famous man who had not achieved his personal ideal.

If the line of Personality is less strong than the Fate line (Plate XI), there is a danger that the material affairs of life, or possibly ill-health, will prevent the full expression of the personality,

97   H

and a sense of being thwarted by Fate will intervene and endanger the contentment of the mind. There seems generally to be some sort of antagonism or struggle for supremacy between the two, the ego and its circumstances, signified by the two lines of Fate and of Personality. It is natural enough— seeing that throughout the world of the living, the individual has to struggle with the environment— that there should also be a struggle in the very centre of conscious life— the human mind. On the whole, I conclude that it is a good indication that the line of Fate should be stronger at the base of the hand than the line of Personality; for I have often seen it so marked in the hands of clever and successful people. As a rule, a strong line of this kind is broken before it reaches the line of Reason; and the line of Personality supplants it as the chief upright line in the hand. I have been told by some whose hands I have read that this exactly represents the past development of their lives. Being talented men and women, they had chafed at the restrictions of their early circumstances (environment); and about the date indicated had been able to override them and assert their own personal aims. In considering the past, they agreed that it was a good thing they had been held back as it were from an impetuous start in early life. Therefore we may perhaps regard a strong beginning of the Fate line as in all probability a good sign, unless it continues to indicate a thwarting of the personal development beyond the line of Reason.

The line of Personality, beginning in or near the eminence of Imagination, as it generally does, indicates that the personality is built up on the imaginative ideas of the self or ego and not on the dictates of others or the circumstances of life.

A good line tending towards a strong index finger shows a desire for power or fame, and the promise of success.

Tending towards the middle finger it points to success in the pursuit of intellectual studies, or of material affairs.

Tending towards the ring finger it is an indication of success in Art, in a talented hand ; or of riches and social success in a practical or a materialistic hand. It may mean a love marriage in an idealistic hand ; more especially if there are two lines running side by side and uncrossed.

Tending towards the little finger it is a sign of success in science, business or politics. A good line running towards one finger with a branch line to another would show the desire of the self

99

for the success of both the abilities indicated. Thus the print of Gladstone's hand in " Cheiro's " book shows the line of Personality going towards the index finger (desire for power and leadership) with a strong branch towards the little finger (success in politics).

A line of Personality beginning in or near the Fate line is unusual. It shows that the force of circumstances, and not the imagination, directs the first beginning of the personal development. A good, clear line promises that this will turn out well.

The line beginning somewhat late might mean discouragement to an ardent young spirit, but the line may always grow down. I have several times seen this happen. A good, clear, but late line is a promise that the personality will achieve its own power and expression of itself ; and that is really the important thing ; indeed, the power is already there and may be achieved at a much earlier date than apparently indicated. But the line should be uncrossed in order that one should have a complete assurance that the joy of full expression will be achieved. If there is a strong line with a finer line crossing it, there is some threat to final achievement ; and the individual showing this crossing should be advised to consider well and carefully whether there is not some obstacle that should be overcome—some weakness of love, perhaps, or denial of sacrifice, some inertness or lack of courage. Twice I have seen such lines fade out and together with their obliteration I have noted a success achieved when it had formerly seemed even more than doubtful. Handreading, in one case, by pointing to a danger, enabled the subject to overcome it.

The entire absence of this line need not cause despair in a mind desiring to be, and to express, its ideal self. A woman's hands which I have seen from time to time during the last twenty years, at one time had no line of Personality at all. A hollow palm in this case was a sign of misfortune, which was bravely borne, though there seemed no hope of alleviation or chance for her self-development. Gradually, however, a line of personal success grew, later on became more and more marked, and of late this person has certainly achieved full self-expression and success. After this experience I should consider no hand whatever destitute of all possibility of growing new lines of promise and success.

Several small lines instead of one strongly marked one show a personality that has many different ways of expressing itself, though it may perhaps be lacking in power in any one direction because of its many interests.

A line made up of little pieces but going steadily up the hand shows that the personality is built up more because of outside influences than by reason of a dominating idea of the self. If each new little line begins before the previous one ends, it shows enhancement of personality and success. We have already considered the lines of Initiative, which run up the palm from the line of Instinct. These lines also indicate personal achievement ; but the fact that they start from a line indicative of an instinctive impulse instead of an imaginative idea, shows that personal achievement may have different origins. I have frequently seen such little lines continuing an unbroken beginning, and indicative of the future ; and in one or two cases when the time came the individuals did in fact begin some career, or some new venture in a career, without fully realising how or why they were acting, though they were conscious of a vague sort of compulsion. But the line of Personality generally springs from the eminence of Imagination, and it represents the conscious wish or desire of the person to find expression in a certain definite way. Though often baffled or retarded by circumstances for a time, the ideal is generally achieved, provided this line is well marked.

The nature of Personality is a controversial matter which is greatly disputed, especially in respect of the possibility of its development beyond the inherited constitution by force of will, or intellect. I may accordingly be wrong in so naming this line. But during many years I have observed its meaning and its growth in the hands of individuals who undoubtedly possessed the peculiar quality of mind generally described as Personality; and I feel sure that there is some justification for my use of the term.

CHAPTER XIII

HEALTH AND OTHER LINES

" CHEIRO " describes the line of Health
(Plate XII) as running down the hand from the
base of the little finger to the line of Instinct,
predicting death at the point where the two lines
meet. Desbarolles, on the contrary, describes
the line as going *up* the hand ; but he attaches
such a superfluity of meanings to a long line—
viz., " good health, rich blood, harmony of the
fluids, a grand memory, a good conscience,
probity, and success in affairs "—that he is hardly
to be regarded as a sane and balanced critic
of the evidence that may reasonably be deduced
from the line of Health. Good health may go
with virtue ; but there are also healthy villains
in the world.

" Cheiro's " description is more lucid and
reasonable ; but, as I have always felt that
Handreaders should not be greatly concerned
with predictions regarding the physical health of
the individual, I have not studied the line and its

significance, and so must refer the student to " Cheiro's " book. Entirely to neglect the line, however, is certainly unwise, for it occupies a prominent position in many hands.

The line of Sensitiveness. This line Palmists call " the girdle of Venus," and they generally describe it as indicating debauchery. " Cheiro " thinks this a mistake, and I agree with him ; though I am of opinion that he also gives it too great a significance as indicating an unbalanced or hysterical nature. It would have this meaning only in a very weak or dissolute hand, where it is most unlikely to be found. I have more often seen it in the hands of musicians than of any other artists ; indeed I cannot remember ever having seen a complete line on any but a musical hand, though parts of the line (the beginning and the end) are frequently seen on hands of every sort and shape.

The line of Sensitiveness begins in the cleft between the index and middle fingers (Plate XII), and when completely formed is a semicircle ending near the base of the little finger. It indicates, when the line is clear, a very sensitive mind. In a well-balanced hand this would be a wholly good and useful indication. In a sensuous hand it might imply extra powers of enjoyment, and possibly might lead to excess of sensual pleasures of an artistic sort, but not to what is generally understood by debauchery; for this would be indicated by an over-soft and over-developed eminence of Instinct. This is very unlikely to be found in the same hand as the line of Sensitiveness.

In a weak hand the line would be likely to indicate overstrung nervous sensitivity. In the character indicated by a square or practical hand such extra sensitiveness would be useful. Should there be a good line of Sensitiveness in the hands of a child who shows also artistic tendencies, it would be well to suggest that every opportunity of developing musical tastes and skill should be given to, but not forced on, him.

The Marriage lines (Plate XII). I have found the current interpretations of these so hopelessly wrong that I do not pay any attention to them, except sometimes for the sake of curiosity. They certainly must have some meaning; but it is strange that all Palmists quote them so confidently as indicating marriage.

The lines supposed to indicate children, too, are nearly always wrongly interpreted. I have long since given up telling maiden ladies how many marriages and children they have had;

PLATE XII

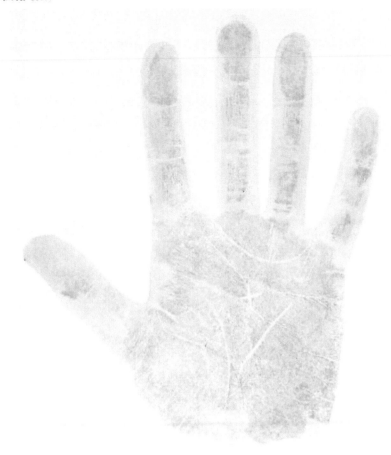

A hand showing the Health line, the Marriage line, the line of Sensitiveness, and the Mystic Cross

though I remember one charming old maid being delighted at the idea that, but for her maidenly pride and reserve, she would have been married twice and have had five children.

The Ring of Solomon forms a semicircle on the base of the index finger. This is another disappointing line. I have never seen it where it could possibly be construed as indicating an "Occult Master." Among the hand prints in "Cheiro's" book, the only one that shows a strong ring of Solomon is the hand of William Whiteley; and there it shows what I believe to be the real significance of the line, namely, a power of ruling and influencing other people. The "Occult Masters" probably possessed this power in an unusual degree and were careful to cultivate it; but it is a mistake to associate the line with any occult or visionary gifts.

Power of obtaining the abstract knowledge of the philosopher, the Vision of the Absolute, or the Mystic Union, would be indicated by the lines of Reason and Intuition, and especially by the formation called by Palmists the Mystic Cross, which is dealt with in the next chapter.

The line of Clairvoyance (Plate III). Palmists call this line that of *Intuition*, but no other name than this is possible for the third primary line; and, having so used it, a new name has to be found for this one. After a special search for individuals who had such a line clearly marked in their hands, and a good deal of study of whatever unusual gifts they undoubtedly possessed, as well as much reading of normal and abnormal psychology, it was clear to me that Clairvoyance was the most suitable name for this interesting line. The word covers the vision of the poet as expressed through his creative ideas, as well as the imaginative perception of the seer or medium whose visions are unhindered by the limits of time and space. I have also seen the line in the left hands of fascinating women, where it indicates the power they possess of intuitive apprehension of the mystery and charm of life.

The line of Clairvoyance when complete forms a sort of half-circle running up the eminence of Imagination and touching or crossing the line of Intuition.

A strongly marked line in a philosophic or intellectual hand indicates a love of visionary ideas. One famous Celtic poet has a strong line of Clairvoyance marked in his left hand.

In a psychic or long, thin hand, the line indicates a power of second sight, or gift of mediumship. By far the best line of Clairvoyance I have ever seen was in the right hand of a famous medium for spirit communication.

In a square hand it is seldom found, but I once observed a fairly good line of Clairvoyance in the hand of an explorer who agreed that he had a curious power of day-dreaming in respect of coming events, and also of seeing through people. He found this very useful in dealing with savage tribes.

In an elementary hand the line rarely occurs, but I once saw a very well-marked one in the hand of a Scotch housemaid who certainly had what she called " the gift."

Parts of this line are often seen in all sorts of hands. They show that the mind has more power of foreseeing events, and seeing through people, than is usual. I am not sure if a broken line can be completed. It seems unlikely, for conscious effort, it would appear, cannot develop the gift of clairvoyance.

CHAPTER XIV

SQUARES, STARS AND CROSSES

Squares indicate preservation from danger, whether to the physical or moral well-being depends on what part of the hand the square is found.

Somewhat reluctantly I have come to the conclusion that a square can be relied on to mean that the individual who exhibits it has had, or will have, some sudden realisation (possibly a barely conscious feeling) that there is a danger of catastrophe, as well as an inspiration of some word, thought or action that will avert it.

Can four little lines in the hand that do not always form a perfect square be significant of such a curious mental process ? This surely must be superstitious nonsense. Truth is truth, however, and I am bound to admit that though I cannot in any rational way account for the significance of the square, yet when clearly formed in the palm it has in my experience proved an indication invariably verified. Some individuals seem to have a sudden foresight that has nothing to do with their ordinary faculties ; it comes to them as a mysterious message from some super-normal power, whether from within the personal unconscious or from beyond it, who shall say ?

A Highland artist, who became a soldier in the Great War, had the strongest and clearest square on the line of Instinct that I have seen, and his explanation was the most vivid I have ever heard.

He had been standing with a small group of other officers at the Front, when he heard :

" Go back and get a cigarette."

He looked round, but no one had spoken. He then heard the voice, seemingly in his own head, say :

" Go back and get a cigarette."   " But I don't want to smoke," he murmured.

" Go back and get a cigarette," came for the third time, and in such an authoritative way that he went back half in a dream.   He returned with the cigarette to find that a shell had burst just where he had been standing.

During the War I was asked to read the hands of a young man of twenty-two who was going out to Gallipoli.   There were no upright lines at all in the palm of his right hand.   I felt this to be an unfavourable sign, as it implied that his mind had no definite plan for the future. Luckily, I was able to assure his mother that the primary lines showed a strong constitution and intelligence, which would no doubt safeguard his life as quick instinctive reactions to danger can frequently avert catastrophe.

For some time after his arrival in the East, there was no news of him. Then a letter came from a hospital in Egypt. He had been badly wounded but was now recovering. Idly looking at his hands one day, he had noticed a curious " square " of lines in the palm of his right hand. He drew a rough sketch of this and, enclosing it in his letter, asked what it meant. I told his mother that all palmists said that a square indicated " preservation from danger " ; and I was quite certain it was not marked in his hand when he went away.

When the young man came home, I asked if I might see the square. It was clearly marked and very noticeable. I questioned the young soldier about his experiences and especially of any particular incident which might explain the square as a warning of danger. He told me that he had been badly wounded in the leg and, unable to walk, was waiting his turn for the stretcher-

bearers who were very busy with desperate cases.
Quite suddenly it flashed into his mind that he
was close to an ammunition dump ; and as shells
were bursting all round it was certain death to
stay where he was. So he just managed to crawl
painfully down to the beach and was then put
on board the hospital ship. In this case I can
swear that there was no sign of a square in his
hand when he went out to the East, and that there
was a very strong one when he came back.
About five years later the square had completely
vanished, but the upright lines in the palm had
grown, showing the development of his mind
and a plan for the future. This case might be
considered trifling by itself, but it is only one of
many where a square in the palm seemed to have
a special significance of danger averted by sudden
foresight.

Once at an evening party I met a group of three
or four interesting men and without knowing
their names or anything about them, looked at
their hands. I was amazed by the strong
" squares " in the palms of their right hands,
which were so much stronger and clearer than
any I had hitherto seen. The men were amused
when I pointed out their " marks of preservation
from danger," and said they had great need of

such protection as they were Antarctic explorers. It was their case that convinced me that squares are worthy of consideration as having a real significance of some unusual mental foresight.

The individual seems to become suddenly aware of a danger signal. This is possibly from some part of the unconscious mind, which, though below the level of consciousness, is capable of the quick, almost uncanny, apprehension of coming events which natives and undeveloped persons often appear to possess in a surprising degree. In their case the conscious realisation is not hindered by intellectual preoccupations.

These are only a few of the many instances I could quote, but they show the mysterious mental processes indicated by the square.

Perhaps we may find among the many meanings Desbarolles gives to a square a hint of its genesis and of the secret power it indicates. In this case he is more analytical than other palmists. He says " a square in the hand announces power, energy of the organ indicated, good sense, justice, seeing at a glance, calm energy." These last two words are suggestive, especially if we slip the word " unconscious " in between them.

Stars are said by Desbarolles to indicate events

over which we have no control, or fatalities. I think, on the contrary, that they indicate events brought about by the strong desire of the mind for that particular event. At any rate that is the explanation that best fits the facts of my experience.

I have seldom seen Stars except on the base of the index finger, and so placed they give the most favourable indication that Stars can give. " Cheiro " says that when it is in the very centre " it promises great honour, power and position ; ambition gratified, and the ultimate success and triumph of the individual." This is rather a load of meaning for one small mark to bear.

I have seen one or two Stars, Crosses, Triangles, etc., as promises that have not yet arrived at the time of their fulfilment, and I am awaiting with interest the dates indicated.

I have not had time or opportunity to give much study to these curious marks, and have not been able to obtain an ancient book which Dr. Vaschide mentions as dealing very fully with them. This is *La Chiromancie Royale,* by Adrian Sicler. But though curious and interesting, these marks may well await investigation until the more valuable and obvious truths of Handreading are established. The Mystic Cross, however, is in a different category ; for strictly speaking its study pertains to that of the primary lines of Reason and Intuition, since these two intellectual capacities are doubly connected by the cross when it is fully formed. In my opinion this means that there are pathways of communication which enable the reason to receive intuitive inspirations more readily than is usual.

The Mystic Cross (Plate XII) *in a good hand* indicates the power of receiving illumination that transcends the ordinary grasp of the intellect. The exact nature of the knowledge thus acquired would depend on the other qualities of the mind, and the vocation or calling of the individual. I imagine that the cross received the name of " Mystic " because it was so frequently seen in the hands of religious individuals who devoted their lives to the service of God and of their fellow men ; and in their case it might well have meant the possibility of that ecstatic moment, called by mystics " the Union," when the soul is at one with God or the Absolute. They then feel what William James points out is essential to the mystical state, *a sense of illumination.* In a lesser degree this would also be felt by individuals engaged in intellectual pursuits, who often speak of the flash of inspiration they sometimes receive. The cross, or some semblance of it, may also be found in elementary hands ; and even the humblest individuals may have flashes of insight. The value of the truth so perceived would, however, depend on the quality of their minds, and might be concerned merely with the ordinary affairs of their lives, so that the term " mystic " does not seem to be always an appropriate name for the cross.

CHAPTER XV

WE have been assuming throughout that the shape, and the occurrence of the lines in the hand is ultimately to be explained by the functioning of centres in the brain.

For the purpose of a scientific examination of Handreading, however, the connection of lines and brain centres is not all-important. It is the correlation between the lines of the hand and the mental characteristics which must be demonstrated. There are new scientific methods employed to-day by which it would be possible to establish this correlation. I understand that by the use of intelligence tests it is now possible to determine the degree of general mental ability possessed by an individual; and by appropriate tests other general functions can also be determined. A person's instinctive propensities and will power, however, are not so easily known, though it is possible to make relative estimates of them. Moreover, by the methods of testing and of estimating, scientists can determine with certainty whether any given quality tends to go with any other by working out their correlations mathematically.

Can these methods be applied to hand-markings ? If so, their correlation with mental characteristics could be proved or disproved with mathematical certainty. For this, the actual measurement of a large number of hands and their markings would be required, together with the reliable estimating of a large number of persons in respect of the different qualities of character and temperament. These data could then be correlated by employing the ordinary statistical formulæ. Surely, it is worth while to do this, possibly by forming a small society or group of persons who could accumulate a sufficiently varied class of hand records, which would then be indexed and arranged.

The modern science of Astronomy has evolved from its earlier and pre-scientific form of Astrology. Alchemy has resulted in Chemistry. The ancient belief in Palmistry may lead to a modern study of the Hand, which might at the same time have scientific value and be of practical use.

The following is a quotation from *The Group Mind*, by Professor McDougall, in which he gives a clear idea of the help such a science of Handreading might afford in the guidance of personal development ; for there is much, as he says, that people never clearly realise with regard to their own minds.

" In the individual mind, even in the most highly developed and self-conscious, the capacities, dispositions and tendencies that make up the whole mind are never fully and adequately present to consciousness ; the individual never knows himself exhaustively, though he may continually progress towards a more complete self-knowledge."

With the aid of Handreading, I believe, the progress of the individual towards self-knowledge, self-control and happiness may be more easily achieved. Making clearer the lessons of the past, and pointing out the hope for the future, may assist in the realisation of the purpose of the mind, and the enhancement of the personality.